"In her book, *Yoga Nidra for Complete Relaxation and Stress Relief*, Julie Lusk masterfully guides us through simple yet exquisite practices whereby we can experience deep relaxation and relief from stress, and experience true health, vitality, resilience, and well-being, wherever we are, whatever our circumstances, throughout our lifetime. I am grateful for the wisdom that Julie offers us through her profoundly accessible, wise, clear, and beautifully written book that reveals the ancient teachings of yoga nidra for both stress relief and healing and restoring our ability to live a peaceful and meaningful life."

> —**Richard Miller, PhD**, clinical psychologist, teacher of meditation, and author of *Yoga Nidra: A Meditative Practice for Deep Relaxation and Healing* and *The iRest Program for Healing PTSD*

"Well researched, clearly written, and authentically lived by the author, Julie Lusk provides the whys, wherefores, and practices for you to reduce and remove stress. The outcome is enhanced health and well-being as life becomes richly and naturally joyful. This book will not only encourage you, it will also guide you to realize the freedom of a full life through yoga nidra."

> —**Joyce Hawkes, PhD**, biophysicist, cell-biologist-turned-healer, and author of *Cell-Level Healing*

"Master hatha yoga teacher Julie Lusk's *Yoga Nidra for Complete Relaxation and Stress Relief* is a stellar book that embraces essential yoga teachings in accessible, clearly written, and practical ways. Her point of view on yoga's ancient wisdom tradition and skill-based practices are wise, fresh, and original. With all the stress in the world, this book and audio set is to be savored—the joy is in the journey!"

> —**Lilias Folan**, known as the "First Lady of Yoga" since her groundbreaking 1972 yoga television series *Lilias, Yoga and You*

"Julie Lusk combines her scrupulous wisdom and skillful technique with decades of compassionate practice to produce this eminently user-friendly book for those seeking practical, portable tools for managing their stress. Her beautiful spirit infuses these pages with a special light that is hers alone. By all means, read, enjoy, and reap the benefits!"

—**Belleruth Naparstek**, author of *Invisible Heroes: Survivors of Trauma and How They Heal*, and creator of the Health Journeys guided imagery audio series

"Drawing on decades of experience as a skilled yoga teacher, Julie Lusk seamlessly integrates ancient Eastern traditions with Western scientific knowledge to provide a clear, practical, step-by-step guide anyone can use to feel less stressed and live a richer, more fulfilling life. Filled with engaging, everyday illustrations, this book illuminates yoga nidra teachings and effectively shows how their principles and practices can help us all become healthier, more balanced, and better integrated—both physically and emotionally."

—**Ronald D. Siegel, PsyD**, part-time assistant professor of psychology at Harvard Medical School, and author of *The Mindfulness Solution: Everyday Practices for Everyday Problems*

"This beautiful book actually radiates the relaxed state it purports to teach! It is a wonderful addition to the yogic canon of resources for finding peace and self-awareness in our lives, and fills an especially needed niche as an approach that does not necessitate the use of strenuous physical postures and practices."

—**Rev. Vidya Vonne, E-RYT 500**, integral yoga teacher trainer at Satchidananda Ashram-Yogaville, Virginia

"*Yoga Nidra for Complete Relaxation and Stress Relief* contains a practical set of spiritual reflections and techniques drawing insights from India's rich yogic traditions. A useful contribution to the growing body of yoga literature for modern-day spiritual seekers, or simply anyone seeking a calmer, more stress-free mode of living."

—**Edwin Bryant, PhD**, professor of Hindu Religion and
Philosophy, Rutgers University

"All relaxation is good. Some is super. Yoga nidra is a superb way to reduce stress and improve your health. I have personally done a variety of yogic exercises for many years and have also done scores of relaxation exercises... I have hundreds of CDs including guided imagery and a great deal of outstanding music. Despite my experience, Julie's *Yoga Nidra for Complete Relaxation and Stress Relief* provides the deepest relaxation I can imagine. If you have not yet conquered the art of relaxation, I strongly recommend her work ASAP!"

—**Norman Shealy, MD, PhD**, neurosurgeon, psychologist,
founding president of the American Holistic Medical
Association, president of Holos Institutes of Health, and
Professor Emeritus of Energy Medicine and President Emeritus
at Holos University Graduate Seminary

"Thank you, Julie, for making the practical and profound practice of yoga nidra clear, concise, and accessible. By first mapping out the effects of stress on body and mind, this book then offers a variety of well-researched relaxation practices to choose from, allowing us the flexibility to choose one or rotate our practice. Relaxation becomes the fertile foundation for living a life that brings us happiness, health, and the dynamic energy to accomplish our heart's dreams. It is a book that would be a welcome addition to any bedside table. That is where my copy will reside!"

—**Nischala Joy Devi**, teacher and author of *The Secret Power
of Yoga* and *The Healing Path of Yoga*

"Congratulations to Julie Lusk on the publication of *Yoga Nidra for Complete Relaxation and Stress Relief*. No question about it—due to the high amount of stress all over and the huge need for a comprehensive anti-stress mechanism, this book is here at just the right time. I feel that this book will definitely help people overcome their stress and other stress-related disorders."

—**Kamakhya Kumar, MSc, PhD (Yogic Science)**, chief editor of *International Journal of Yoga and Allied Sciences*, founding teacher and associate professor in the department of yoga and health, and chief coordinator at the Center of Complementary and Alternative Medicine at Dev Sanskriti University, Haridwar, India

"*Yoga Nidra for Complete Relaxation and Stress Relief* is a very comprehensive study of the positive effects that yoga has on combating the stress and tension we all hold on to. It is a well-organized and very practical guide. The personal stories clearly demonstrate how yoga directly decreases stress and why. The questionnaire is a great tool for personally guiding the reader toward the path of stress reduction. Once our stressors and symptoms are identified, we are more equipped to conquer them. Julie Lusk has created a book that describes the philosophy, physiology, and spirituality of yoga, and directly connects this to stress reduction. It is an extremely valuable and interesting book from beginning to end. I highly recommend it to anyone who is seriously interested in managing the stress both in their personal and professional lives."

—**Don R. Powell, PhD**, president and CEO of the American Institute for Preventive Medicine

"Yoga nidra is a very effective and useful tool to relieve daily stress, to promote deep healing, to reprogram subconscious negative patterns, and to release energy blocks that prevent us from growing physically and spiritually. In this book, Julie Lusk provides a very good and elaborate description of its benefits, how it works, and the technique to practice it. A recommended book for anyone."

—**Krishna Darshan (Alan Wiuker)**, direct disciple of Swami Vishnu-Devananda, teacher of yoga teacher training courses, Vedanta philosophy, and Vedic Astrology at the International Sivananda Ashrams since 1986

"Yoga nidra is the art and science of relaxing consciously and deeply to reveal one's true Self. It streamlines and magnifies the powerful benefits from meditative practice, traditional yoga, and conventional yoga postures by combining the essence of each into one discipline. In a beautiful way, Julie Lusk has brought to our awareness how this powerful synthesis is clearly possible and provides proven methods.... It is as energizing as it is healing."

—**Donna Eden and David Feinstein,** coauthors of *The Energies of Love* and *Energy Medicine*

"Julie Lusk's *Yoga Nidra for Complete Relaxation and Stress Relief* is a beautiful and effective guide to a most important practice for our times. Based on the philosophy that inner peace is not something we must construct but rather discover within ourselves, it inspires spiritual as well as psychological healing. I highly recommend this book to anyone seeking relief from our modern epidemic of stress."

—**Rubin Naiman, PhD**, clinical assistant professor of Medicine at the University of Arizona Center for Integrative Medicine, Clinical and Sleep Health Psychology, and director of Circadian Health Associates

"What a delight to have access to such a comprehensive book and audio files on yoga nidra. As a practitioner and teacher with decades of experience, I appreciate information that not only serves me but also my students. Hats off to Julie Lusk, a remarkable woman, teacher, friend, and author."

—**Vandita Kate Marchesiello, E-RYT 500**, teacher and faculty member at Kripalu Center for Yoga and Health, and recording artist on the best-selling CDs *Transform, Relax, and Rejuvenate, Yoga with Vandita,* and *Vandita Chants*

"Offering anecdotal and scientific evidence, interactive stress assessment tools, scripts, and free downloadable audio practices, *Yoga Nidra for Complete Relaxation and Stress Relief* is an important contribution to the literature on yoga and mental health. Julie Lusk's clear, calm writing and speaking voice offers a balm for the troubled mind. What I love most about practicing with Julie is that her practices are progressive, gentling us into the deeper work of significant and beneficial change."

—**Amy Weintraub**, founder of LifeForce Yoga Healing Institute, and author of *Yoga for Depression* (Broadway Books) and *Yoga Skills for Therapists* (W. W. Norton)

"Along with biofeedback and meditation, the practice of yoga has garnered increasing interest and application in the management of stress and trauma. In her new book, *Yoga Nidra for Complete Relaxation and Stress Relief*, Julie Lusk provides both a comprehensive review of the rationale and practice of yoga nidra, and a beautifully developed, step-by-step manual for its effective practice. She presents a comprehensive, lay-friendly review of the body-brain physiology of stress, which provides a powerful scientific background for its practice. This is an important addition to the literature on the management of health and the treatment of chronic disease and trauma."

—**Robert C. Scaer, MD**, author of *The Body Bears the Burden: Trauma, Dissociation, and Disease, The Trauma Spectrum,* and *Eight Keys to Brain-Body Balance*

"Julie Lusk, an experienced yoga teacher, has written a very thorough book not only on yoga nidra—*to sleep into union with oneself*—but also on the whole topic of stress and relaxation. Offering important research as to why relaxation is important, she then takes us step-by-step through invaluable exercises and meditations to reconnect us to our inner joy and peace. This book is suitable for all those who are ready to take the stress out of life."

—**Christine Page, MD**, teacher and author of *Frontiers of Health*

"*Yoga Nidra for Complete Relaxation and Stress Relief* provides a positive set of self-help tools that can be used by anyone, almost anywhere, and most anytime. I have successfully used Julie's curriculum and recordings both personally and professionally. Students report feeling relaxed, safe, and clear, and grounded and refreshed with vibrant energy. Her methodology and instructions contribute to reductions in stress, anxiety, and negative thinking. Julie's systematic analysis of stress, inclusion of research, and references to evidence-based studies add scientific credibility to this yogic process and beautifully complement the thousands of years of traditional anecdotal evidence that repeatedly demonstrate the efficacy of this subtle, highly sophisticated approach to mind-body well-being. This book is an essential resource for anyone interested in developing greater self-reliance for their own well-being and to have enhanced capacity to be of genuine service to others."

—**Christopher Baxter**, architect, yoga educator, and author of *Kripalu Hatha Yoga*

"Julie's wonderful book, *Yoga Nidra for Complete Relaxation and Stress Relief*, is exactly that. It allows the reader to be aware and identify stress and to mindfully treat and control its effects with the use of yoga nidra. The power of using *sankalpas*, *koshas*, and *mudras* is clearly explained and empowers the effectiveness of yoga nidra. The technique of yoga nidra is easily understood, safe, and practical, and truly a great resource for anyone, especially those seeking relief from the effects of stress as well as helping professionals of all types who provide stress management to others."

—**June Greenwood**, proprietor of Redcliffe Yoga Centre in Redcliffe, Queensland, Australia

"Many people think of yoga as physical poses and stretching. While these are a part of yoga, I learned in my first yoga teacher training over twenty years ago that yoga nidra is the most important part of a practice—especially for stressed-out people. I really appreciate the way Julie provides context, scientific data, and practical applications. Whether you are new to yoga or are a longtime practitioner, yoga nidra will enhance and expand your practice and transform your life."

—**Deborah Kern, PhD (Health Sciences)**, Integral Hatha Yoga Instructor, Black Belt Nia Instructor, and Phoenix Rising Yoga Therapist

"Yoga nidra is a much-needed antidote to our fast-paced living, balancing the rapid vinyasa practices that have taken over the yoga world. Clear and concise, this book embodies the true essence of yoga, which is about cultivating a state of aware stillness. From this place, the jewels of consciousness can arise. With step-by-step instructions, well grounded in yoga philosophy, this book outlines a practice that could change your life. Julie Lusk has written a real gem."

—**Anodea Judith, PhD**, author of *Eastern Body, Western Mind* and *Wheels of Life*

"Julie Lusk skillfully guides us through the accessible and inviting practice of yoga nidra, a powerful practice to transform our stressed-out, modern-day life. Because yoga nidra leads you through the five levels of being (*koshas*), it is the most thoroughly relaxing of all meditations. Julie's book is a warm invitation for everyone, from all walks of life, to enjoy and benefit from the true deep relaxation that yoga nidra can give!"

—**Jennifer Reis, E-RYT 500**, faculty member at Kripalu Center for Yoga and Health and Integrative Yoga Therapy, and creator of Divine Sleep Yoga Nidra® and Five Element Yoga®

"Julie's done it again. Because she walks her talk, her work is authentic and able to take you to deeper parts of yourself. I recommend this book to all."

—**John W. Travis, MD**, coauthor of *Wellness Workbook*

"Julie Lusk is a true professional in the field of mind-body healing. *Yoga Nidra for Complete Relaxation and Stress Relief* explores the various dimensions of this ancient and practical science, showing us why we need yoga nidra, along with an in-depth understanding of how it works. This book is a must for all of us who need to relax!"

—**Joseph Le Page**, founder and director of Integrative Yoga Therapy, faculty member at Kripalu Center for Yoga and Health since 1996, and founder and director of Enchanted Mountain Center in Brazil, the largest yoga retreat in South America

"Julie Lusk takes us on a profound journey into our deeper beings, bringing us to an inner peace and calm. She offers concrete steps for living stress-free, which can change our whole experience of life forever! Julie has the great gift for helping us enter that peaceful space where we live and act from our 'True Self'—living a life of meaning and joy.... This book not only gives us hope that it is possible to live a stress-free life, full of joy and meaning—it also shows us how to do it!"

—**Elaine Valdov, PhD**, psychotherapist and activist, representative to the United Nations, president and founder of Yogis Beyond Borders/Yoga Peace Ambassadors and International Young Leaders Vision Summits

"I've found Julie Lusk to be a fount of practical knowledge on yoga, meditation, and stress management since I first met her more than twenty years ago. Whether you are new to conscious relaxation or a long-term yoga practitioner, this book offers a comprehensive, user-friendly, and stress-busting approach to yoga nidra. It is grounded in classical yoga, backed by contemporary science, and features easy-to-follow instructions you can start practicing right now to bring you into balance and turn on your healing faculties. *Yoga Nidra for Complete Relaxation and Stress Relief* can change the way you deal with stress forever."

—**Danna Faulds**, author of six books of poetry and the memoir *Into the Heart of Yoga: One Woman's Journey*

"I love this book! *Yoga Nidra for Complete Relaxation and Stress Relief* will dramatically change your beliefs about yourself, your health, and your life! Julie Lusk knows the deeper practices and inner truths of yoga and shares them in understandable and informative ways. As a naturopathic physician, I listen to patients diagnosed with life-threatening diseases and often hear the inner conflict between their subconscious and conscious beliefs. Resolving these conflicts, and thus dramatically changing their health, is vital. Yoga nidra, and using a *sankalpa*, is designed to accomplish this."

—**Judy Fulop, ND, FABNO**

"*Yoga Nidra for Complete Relaxation and Stress Relief* by Julie Lusk is chock-full of practical exercises that anyone can use to get started in a regular meditation practice. From short relaxation, breathing, and meditation options to guided imagery, Lusk gives you the tools you'll need to develop greater resiliency so that you can overcome physical, mental, and emotional stress."

—**Ruth Buczynski, PhD**, licensed psychologist, and president of the National Institute for the Clinical Application of Behavioral Medicine

"Once again Julie Lusk provides us with practical tools to help us find relaxation, meaning, and purpose in an increasingly stressful world. *Yoga Nidra for Complete Relaxation and Stress Relief* offers a great mix of self-management skills and personal anecdotes from Julie's three decades as an educator and yoga instructor. Everyone will benefit from this extremely timely book and refer to it often as a way to find their way back to a path toward a more peaceful and joyful life."

—**Dan Bernstein**, president of Personal Health Designs

"*Yoga Nidra for Complete Relaxation and Stress Relief* is a must-read to balance out the stress of modern times. Lusk's writing is engaging, easy to read, and easy to understand, and makes stress relief practices desirable and accessible for everyday life."

—**Luna Ray**, teacher of yoga, workshop and retreat leader, kirtan musician and recording artist, and advocate for conscious and empowered community collaboration

# Yoga Nidra
## *for* Complete Relaxation & Stress Relief

**Julie Lusk,** MEd, E-RYT

New Harbinger Publications, Inc.

## Publisher's Note

*Yoga Nidra for Complete Relaxation and Stress Relief* is geared to help stressed-out people. Yoga Nidra is not a replacement for appropriate medical care. It can be used to reduce symptoms, side effects, and help with your ability to cope with your issues. If you have a serious medical condition or mental illness, consult your health care providers to get their advice before proceeding and to supervise your health status as your practice progresses.

Distributed in Canada by Raincoast Books

"Inner Light" from PRAYERS TO THE INFINITE: NEW YOGA POEMS by Danna Faulds; copyright © 2004 Danna Faulds. "Where Inquiry and Knowing Meet" and "This Is What I Have to Say to You" from BREATH OF JOY: POEMS, PRAYERS, AND PROSE by Danna Faulds; copyright © 2013 Danna Faulds. Reprinted by permission of the author.

The kubera mudra, hakini mudra, and ishvara mudra illustrations that appear in appendix 1 of this book are reprinted with permission from MUDRAS FOR HEALING AND TRANSFORMATION by Joseph Le Page and Lilia Le Page. Copyright © 2013 Joseph Le Page and Lilia Le Page. Reprinted by permission of Integrative Yoga Therapy.

The "Alternate Nostril Breathing" and "Cultivate the Positive" practices in appendix 2 of this book and the whole of appendix 4 have been adapted from YOGA MEDITATIONS by Julie Lusk. Copyright © 2005 Julie Lusk. Used by permission of Whole Person Associates.

Copyright © 2015 by Julie Lusk

      New Harbinger Publications, Inc.
      5674 Shattuck Avenue
      Oakland, CA 94609
      www.newharbinger.com

Cover design by Amy Shoup; Acquired by Wendy Millstine; Edited by Marisa Solís

### Library of Congress Cataloging-in-Publication Data

Lusk, Julie T.
  Yoga nidra for complete relaxation and stress relief / Julie Lusk, MEd, NCC, E-RYT.
    pages cm
  Includes bibliographical references.
  ISBN 978-1-62625-182-3 (paperback) -- ISBN 978-1-62625-183-0 (pdf e-book) -- ISBN 978-1-62625-184-7 (epub) 1. Hatha yoga. 2. Relaxation. 3. Stress management. I. Title.
  RA781.7.L87 2015
  613.7'046--dc23

                    2015005459

Printed in the United States of America

21    20    19

10   9   8   7   6   5   4

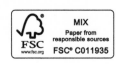

MIX
Paper from responsible sources
FSC
www.fsc.org    FSC® C011935

# Where Inquiry and Knowing Meet

Acknowledge the body,
acknowledge the mind,
embrace the relative realm
with all the energy and
gusto you can find—
just don't stop there.
Behind, beneath, beyond
sensory experience and
identity is the silent
spacious yes of your
true nature. Now I'm
not saying that this
world isn't real,
but there's more to you
than what you think,
taste, see, or feel.
Choose the whole,
and not the part.
Choose the fire, not
the spark. Acknowledge
your heart, but identify
only with what's infinite
and free, and eventually
let even that fall away
to leave the open space
where inquiry and
knowing meet as equals.

—Danna Faulds

# Contents

# Acknowledgments

I am brimming with gratitude for the opportunity to give you this book and these audio files, and I appreciate all those, seen and unseen, who have lent a helping hand.

This all got started when Krishna Darshan (Alan Wiuker) read my Vedic astrology chart while I was teaching at the Sivananda Ashram Yoga Retreat in the Bahamas. My skepticism slowly started fading when he described me better than my parents could. He said that opportunities were coming my way that would expand my reach in the area of writing, giving workshops, and teaching in general. "Yoga nidra," he said—a topic I have been studying, practicing, and teaching for decades—"fit right into my chart." Imagine the look on my face when Wendy Millstine, an acquisitions editor for New Harbinger Publications, sent me an e-mail a few months later to ask if I was interested in writing a book on yoga nidra. The doubts I had about Krishna's forecast vanished into thin air.

You are the recipient of this fascinating phenomenon. May you reap untold benefits through experiencing yoga nidra for complete relaxation and stress relief.

My loving appreciation goes to my husband, Dave, who describes himself as "the common man." In other words, someone with an unlimited experience with stress and a limited understanding of yoga. His encouragement and support were endless. He seemed to know exactly when I needed breaks and when not to interrupt; he kept me laughing and prepared lots of delicious food that kept me happy and healthy. He often stopped what he was busy with to listen to me read chapters and exercises to him, and to offer his feedback and comments. He started out thinking that relaxation was a stupid waste of time and changed into asking for more experiences. All of us benefit from his insights and advice.

I have enormous gratitude for all my teachers and am pleased to share their knowledge with you. In particular, let me thank Lilias Folan, Nischala Joy Devi, Joseph and Lilian Le Page, Christopher Baxter, Richard Miller, Amy Weintraub, Saraswati Neumann, Kamakhya Kumar, Joe Panoor, and all those at Integral Yoga, Sivananda Yoga, Kripalu Center for Yoga and Health, Inner Sky Yoga, and White Lotus.

A great deal of what I learn comes from those who have attended my classes, retreats, and workshops and gladly offered their time to experience yoga nidra, experimented with resolves by using a sankalpa, and shared their stories. Please keep it up.

My heart goes out to all my friends who cheered me on, gave me room to write, and offered me much-needed breaks that were fun and refreshing. I especially want to thank Elizabeth TenOever, Beth Coulson, Ray and Anna Vasudevan, Susanne Quigley, Albert Bollinger, Tara Laurie Moon, Beth Owens, Linda McCachran Brown, Noreen Wessling, Amy Orr, Cindy Lewis, Heather Hurley, Karen Sawyer, Kyra Back, and Arpi Anderson. Sophie and Lucy, our dogs, kept me company and reminded me to go outside to enjoy the fresh air and their antics. My heartfelt love and appreciation is always with the Nichols family, especially my sister, Mary Noel.

Generous contributions of information, ideas, and technical support were made by Christopher Baxter, Danna Faulds, Nischala Joy Devi, Laura K. Strachan, Caroline West, Rev. Saraswati Neumann, Kris Gentry, John Sawyer, Lynn Somerstein, and Carlene Sippola at Whole Person Associates. Joseph and Lilian Le Page gladly contributed the graphics of the mudras. Maynard Chapman expertly illustrated the motor cortex and the model of the koshas as a labyrinth.

The team at New Harbinger Publications stood beside me every step of the way. Their brilliant suggestions and magnificent support have brought amazing layers of depth to *Yoga Nidra for Complete Relaxation and Stress Relief*. Everybody was easy to work with, knowledgeable, and organized. Those who worked with me directly were Wendy Millstine, Jess O'Brien, Jess Beebe, Nicola Skidmore, Vicraj Gill, Marisa Solís, Angela Autry Gorden, and Michele Waters. Thanks to all the countless others who worked behind the scenes to make this project a reality.

Many thanks to Jeanne Fredericks, my literary agent, who is exceptionally smart, thoughtful, and kind.

Please join me in giving everyone a huge smile and a standing ovation. Toot, toot!

# Introduction

"I can't remember a time in my life that wasn't stressful. Through the years, I had many difficult moments raising children, dealing with my husband's bipolar disorder and ADHD, holding down a job, and staying on top of household chores. I used to think that stress helped me get things done, but I was wrong. All that stress caught up with me with an assortment of illnesses and problems. Practicing yoga nidra at my weekly yoga class and listening to a recording nightly has made a huge difference for me. I now have the tools to take care of myself throughout my day and continually encourage others to do the same. I finally learned to breathe correctly, and I practice breathing everywhere. Tensing and releasing tight muscles helps calm me down. I've learned to quit grinding my teeth and be more mindful of what is going on inside me, to take time to heal and let go of what I can't control. My class gives me joy. Yoga is my salvation."

—Debbie, hospital lab technician

Did you know that yoga can be practiced without performing physical exercises? Were you aware that meditation can be done lying down instead of sitting up still and straight like a statue? What if doing so gave you a personal understanding of the core principles of yoga and resulted in living happily, peacefully, and with meaning and purpose—*without stress*? Yoga nidra (pronounced *nih-drah*) is the way.

To live happy, healthy, and fulfilling lives, we must learn to live in harmony with life in the midst of stressful conditions as well as enjoy the good times. Yoga nidra has exactly what it takes to accomplish this because it combines the profound principles and practices of yoga's wisdom teachings with powerful mindbody techniques. Yoga nidra systematically and effectively combines the best of stress management, relaxation training, guided imagery, and meditation. It has practical tools you can use for quick relief when bombarded by stress, teaches ways to prevent reacting to stress inappropriately, and gives long-lasting results. It is relaxing, reflective, and revitalizing.

You *can* experience stress relief right away. There is no need to know anything about yoga to gain these benefits. All you have to do is practice the yoga nidra exercises. Practicing each exercise as a whole is recommended in the beginning to get the full effect. Just the same, focusing on the segments that you prefer is quite helpful, especially if time is short. The time needed ranges from minutes to up to an hour. While attending yoga nidra classes is helpful and enjoyable, there is no need to do so. Using this book and the free audio downloads that accompany it are enough. Ongoing practice will enable you to integrate the skills being taught into your daily life for not only combating stress but to feel more energized and at ease. Stressful worries will be transformed by developing a sensible and wise source of inner guidance.

Yoga nidra is not a religion. People from all faith traditions and religious backgrounds can and do benefit. Most find that it supports their religious convictions in genuine ways.

One step at a time, *Yoga Nidra for Complete Relaxation and Stress Relief* will give you the understanding and experiential exercises needed to genuinely dissolve stress into inner peacefulness and joy with the experience of profound contentment and wholeness. Physical comfort and relaxation is experienced, mental and emotional distress is minimized, limiting beliefs are lessened, and intuitive awareness and wisdom blossom to guide our perceptions, interpretations, and actions. These qualities become more available throughout the day the more we dwell in the yoga nidra state of consciousness.

The stories in this book are told by people who want to share with you how yoga nidra has helped reduce their stress and been of benefit to them. They are told in their own words. Perhaps you can relate to what some of them have to say:

"Deciding to change careers was a difficult move in my life. I knew in my heart it was what I needed to do, but it left me feeling very much alone. I tend to overthink and overanalyze everything, so my big challenge was in giving my mind a rest—it tended to be *very* anxious. I remember doing yoga nidra for the first time and feeling so calm and still. My mind had focus, and I was 100 percent worry-free. It was easy to experience *being in the moment*, and the instructions for doing so were easy to follow. Spending time doing yoga nidra has a carryover effect to my general well-being. The calm center of peace remains. I feel refreshed and ready to meet whatever or whoever comes my way. Above all, it helps to still my overly anxious mind. I have the tools needed for bringing on restful peace that is so good for my body and mind. In turn, it helps me have better relationships. Yoga nidra is wonderful—it is a gift!"

—Laura, high school teacher

"I was recovering from a broken hand and was very stressed by the length of the recovery. During a yoga nidra session, I felt like my whole skeleton was trying to tell me something in a message. As this continued, I began to feel my body slow down and my stress level begin to decrease. I also discovered that the breathing techniques are great for dealing with pain and stress. I am sleeping better."

—Mary, elected municipal government official

"Starting retirement was very stressful. There were so many unknowns, and I was really worried about my finances. Yoga nidra helped me begin to think differently and to enjoy each day. I am able to deal with changes calmly, and the pain in my abdomen went away. I feel better about myself because I am now prioritizing myself."

—Ann, retired financial planner

## Stress and Its Impact

Stress is everywhere these days. No one is immune. Stressors comes in all shapes, sizes, and circumstances—from traffic jams to terminal illness. In addition to outside stressors, the way we think and the way we react can cause undue stress. Worry, concern for oneself and others, and mistaken beliefs can fire up feelings of stress in no time at all.

Stress is motivating when it inspires us to meet a deadline and do our best. When handled poorly, it can cause problems ranging from mild irritation to devastation. Stressed-out people suffer from aches and pains of all types, fatigue, feeling nervous, racing thoughts, sleeplessness, indecision, impatience, and fear, to name a few. Stress affects home and work life, and robs us of peace of mind. It either causes or contributes to the vast majority of illnesses and can take the pleasure out of life.

Many falsely believe that one can achieve stress relief by simply watching television or checking social media sources, or by drinking or eating too much. These are distractions from tension and *not* true stress relief. Unfortunately, too many people don't refresh themselves by taking enough time to completely relax and recuperate.

Stress is powerful, but so is relaxation training. *Real relaxation is more than something nice to do if there is time. It is an essential life skill!* Yoga nidra is relaxation at its finest and puts the meaning back into living.

"I internalize stress: stress from work, from family, from myself— faults, insecurities, weakness. This makes me impatient, intolerant, and mean, and I don't like myself when I get this way.

Yoga nidra has brought me to a peaceful place. I am able to tap my inner strength and beauty."

—Kathy, mother and public relations specialist

"Workplace stress used to eat me up. I was afraid of not measuring up, I felt pressure from my bosses, and there wasn't enough time to complete tasks efficiently. I'm certain that without yoga nidra I would have gone bonkers. It helps me stay alert, present, and nonreactive. The fear does not possess me when it visits anymore. I am much more comfortable at work events and social settings."

—Beth, construction manager

Chapter 1 will give you the details you need to understand stress, its consequences, and what you can do about it. The Assess Your Stress questionnaire will help you identify your stressors to enable you to concentrate your stress-relieving efforts effectively.

## Yoga's Solutions for Stress Relief

As is stress, yoga seems to be everywhere too. More than 20 million people practice in the United States alone. In modern times, yoga has become almost synonymous with going to a class and doing postures, maybe trying out some specialized yoga breathing, and, at the end, resting for a short time before class is over. This is fortunate because the physical aspect of yoga has remarkable benefits. Having practiced and taught postures and breathing since the mid-seventies, I have seen it relieve stress and its consequences over and over in people of all ages and fitness levels. With practice, their coping skills increase and energy lifts. People often become more physically fit and mentally stable, and their emotions smooth out. Scientists are confirming what ancient yogis knew all along: the mind and body are one, and yoga is healing for the body, mind, and spirit.

It is exciting that millions of practicing yogis and the general public are now realizing that yoga is much more than physical postures. Yoga nidra is the perfect solution for those who want to take their experience of doing postures to a deeper level and magnify its healing and life-enriching benefits. Furthermore, it provides a yogic path and method to people who long for the benefits of yoga but are not interested in or capable of practicing yoga postures.

Meditation is also growing in popularity. Like yoga, it is being taught in medical settings, schools, community centers, at the workplace, and where people worship. This is all being fueled by the results people are gaining and the research behind it. Yoga nidra makes the meditation process easier, enjoyable, and deeply rewarding. Instead of having to sit as in meditation, it is usually done lying down. We will see in chapter 2 how yoga nidra is an important link that bridges the practice of yoga postures with meditation and thereby enhances both.

Guided imagery—the positive and relaxing use of one's mind and imagination—is being used for relaxation, personal growth, and for health improvement. The site http://www.healthjourneys.com offers a compendium of hundreds of studies that document the healing nature of guided imagery for a host of medical conditions such as insomnia, depression, panic attacks, hypertension, and post-traumatic stress, to name a few. Guided imagery has been practiced as part of yoga nidra for ages and is called *bhavana*.

> "My mother died a few years ago. My heart ached for the love only a mother can give. One evening during yoga nidra, I had an experience I will never forget. Lying on my mat completely relaxed and breathing softly and rhythmically, I felt as if I were being hugged on the inside in my heart area. I felt a connection with my mother that was emotional, physical, and spiritual all at the same time. Intuitively, I knew this hug had come from my mother, and it filled me with joy and wonder knowing that her loving spirit continues on. Yoga nidra allowed me to experience her love and her hug again in a very real way."
>
> —Sue, social worker and therapist

## Yoga Nidra in a Nutshell

Yoga nidra is a powerful form of yoga that has been practiced for thousands of years as a process of awakening to one's true Self.* "Yoga nidra" means "yogic sleep" and goes far beyond deep relaxation to a place of natural peace and quiet that is tremendously healing. The first stage of relaxation brings about a calm mind while the body feels heavy and deeply relaxed. An inner stillness is also felt during the second stage. As relaxation progresses, the heaviness lifts and a light, buoyant feeling arises. It is somewhat like lingering in the interval between being awake and asleep. Eventually, you will be able to remain alert and aware with a spacious, timeless feeling that is extremely peaceful while your mind and body sleep.

Specialized relaxation exercises, breathing techniques, meditation, and guided imagery are utilized for becoming extremely relaxed and to replenish energy. The unique experience of complete awareness without words, thoughts, images, feelings, and other sensations is felt. It takes you to a place where your innate wisdom, intelligence, and intuition naturally reside. Yoga nidra effectively handles everyday tension and is capable of healing deep-seated stress. It is much more than a quick fix.

One of the main tenets of Yoga philosophy is that *each and every one of us has an indestructible center that is already peaceful, joyful, wise, soulful, luminous, and loving.* This "center" is referred to as the *Atma (individual soul)* or Atman (universal soul) and is believed to be our true Self.

By nature of being human, the Atma is covered up by layers that the Yoga sages call *koshas* (pronounced KOH-shahs). These layers, or sheaths, are physical, energetic, mental-emotional, intuitive, and joyful. While each of these aspects is needed to be alive and well, it is easy to get distracted with the misunderstanding that they are real and permanent. This causes us to lose the capacity to feel authentic contentment, and we can fail to recognize and fulfill our own ultimate meaning and purpose of life on Earth.

---

* "Self" with a capital "S" refers to one's authentic identity, or Atma, whereas "self" with a lowercase "s" refers to our human nature and all our roles.

Yoga masters believe that stress management and relaxation training are valuable. However, it is thought that stress will always be experienced, at least to some extent, until we can eventually identify with our true Self. This amazing, life-changing realization happens gradually. Yoga nidra gives us the direct experience that *our inner core is stress-free* and that *unshakable inner peace and joy really exist within rather than outside ourselves.* We learn firsthand about the temporary nature of our thoughts, feelings, and emotions, and this changes our perspective on stress and on ourselves. Our own personal faith and beliefs, religious or otherwise, are supported, clarified, and enhanced. This gives us the ability to truly quiet our mind, open our heart with compassion, and do some real healing for high-level living. Everyday stresses are handled much more easily. These concepts will be explored further in chapter 2.

> "I have the generic stress of a woman in her forties: a house, husband, kids, parents, career. I am the one who lives in the middle of the huge web, and I feel that I'm the one who has to keep each string exactly at the right tension so that the whole thing doesn't collapse. I cherish yoga nidra time. It is one of the few times I am totally relaxed and in touch with myself. When most deeply relaxed, I feel like I am floating. After it's over, I feel refreshed, awake, calm, centered, and ready for the rest of my day and week."
>
> —Nancy, working parent

> "I'm taking care of my mother, who has Alzheimer's disease. It's very draining and tiring. Yoga nidra takes me to another place, where I feel like I'm floating without a care. I get my energy back and feel at ease again."
>
> —BevySue, yoga teacher

> "Yoga nidra and its component parts enable me to know that I can depend on myself, especially during my most stressful times."
>
> —Kris, real estate appraiser

## Benefits of Yoga Nidra

With regular practice, your physical and mental health will surely improve as stress diminishes. Yoga nidra changes your physical and emotional responses to stress in the short term and for the long run. You will gain a fresh perspective, enabling you to remain calm and in control—even in the midst of chaos. Chapter 2 documents yoga nidra's known benefits. For now, know that yoga nidra can boost your immune system, decrease inflammation, and reduce pain. Symptom relief related to cancer, asthma, diabetes, addictions, heart disease, and migraine headaches can happen when it is used in conjunction with conventional medical care. Yoga nidra can be used to control physical body functions such as breathing, heart rate, blood pressure, metabolism, body temperature, and even brain waves. Though it's not a substitute for sleeping, one hour of yoga nidra equals about four hours of typical sleep, because the brain wave states we go through (beta, alpha, theta, and delta) are extremely restful and relaxing.

You'll enjoy living with a clear head. Bouncing back from mood swings and emotional upsets gets faster and easier. Your creativity and intuition will flourish in a positive and productive way. Plus, your energy increases.

The brain wave state we're in during yoga nidra is fertile ground. We're both very relaxed and very receptive. Setting a resolve (*sankalpa*) during this time makes it completely possible to clear out useless habits and bring about positive and permanent changes in your personality and life. Chapter 3 goes into detail about what a sankalpa is and how to use one, and these skills are practiced and put to the test in the exercises found in chapters 4 through 6 and in the audio downloads.

"I chose 'I am healthy' as my sankalpa during my summer break from teaching. I wanted to have physical health as well as healthy thoughts and attitudes. Ultimately, my sankalpa influenced me to eat better, exercise more, and be aware of my thoughts and feelings. Yet at first I had doubts that the sankalpa was having an impact. But when I returned to school, I noticed a big difference right away. I was having my best year teaching in fifteen years!

Things just weren't bothering me like they had in the past. Most telling was that fellow teachers also noticed—they asked what was different about me, what I had done over summer break. I gladly told them that I started adding yoga nidra with a sankalpa to my regular practice of yoga postures. I recommended that they try it. And guess what? Several colleagues have followed my lead!"

—Pat, teacher

Yoga nidra can go way beyond stress relief and into the realm of Self-realization and the meeting of the true Self. Patanjali, known as a scientist and philosopher, is considered to be the father of Yoga and author of the *Yoga Sutras* (200 BCE). The *Yoga Sutras* are composed of 196 lines that sum up the practical philosophy of Yoga. They were originally written in Sanskrit and have been translated into other languages over the years by many authors. Each author tries to do his or her best to interpret what Patanjali wanted to get across. This book will typically use the Sanskrit terms, since English interpretations often cannot convey the full meaning originally intended. In addition, becoming familiar with the Sanskrit will make it easier for you to delve deeper into the yogic literature for more information about these concepts.

Yoga Sutra I.2 says, "Yoga is the settling of the mind into silence" (Shearer 1982, 90) and the "uniting of consciousness in the heart" (Devi 2007, 12). Through all my years of practice, study, and teaching others, I have not found a more effective or reliable method of stilling the mind, healing and restoring the body, understanding and managing emotions, and awakening the spirit. High-level health and wellness often occur. There is more to living life than handling stress. It's about living a life of meaning and purpose (*dharma*) and ultimately reaching Self-realization (*atma-jnana*). Yoga nidra gives us a pathway and method for doing so—and it feels wonderful.

"I sleep much better after yoga nidra. I have more energy and mental focus too. It takes me to a place of inner self-awareness, almost like when I was a child, my inner child, who I really am."

—Judy, office administrator

"My stresses caused me not to breathe properly. Yoga nidra relaxed me into a place of the divine. It connected me to my Father in heaven and the Father of all. My stress disappeared and I found my bliss."

—April, self-employed

## How to Use this Book

To summarize, chapter 1 gives you a good understanding of stress. The Assess Your Stress questionnaire will help identify how stress impacts you. Have a notebook or journal handy for jotting down your answers and for notes on your progress. Chapters 2 and 3 cover what yoga nidra is all about and how to practice it. Three yoga nidra methods with variations are provided in written form in chapters 4 through 6. Reading the material provides you with the solid foundation and motivation needed to understand yoga nidra, but to get the maximum benefits, it is essential to experience it firsthand. You have access to free audio downloads of the main exercises available in this book, since it would be difficult to read along and do the yoga nidra practices simultaneously. If you're ready to experience yoga nidra right away, go ahead and jump right in with the practices. You can always go back and pick up the information you skipped. After a while, you will be able to use these new skills for stress relief when necessary and without needing the book or audio.

Additional breathing exercises, other supplemental practices, hand gestures called yoga *mudras*, short relaxation techniques and meditations, and how to lead yoga nidra for others are offered in the appendices to complement your experience.

## How to Download Your Free Audio

To download the audio files that accompany this book, open your browser and go to http://www.newharbinger.com/31823. Follow the instructions provided online.

Additional guided relaxation, imagery, and meditation recordings and books by Julie Lusk are available at http://www.wholesomeresources .com.

Listening to recorded meditations and guided exercises may cause drowsiness. Please do not do so while driving a motor vehicle or operating machinery.

Enjoy!

## Welcome to Yoga Nidra

Good luck and have fun as you delve into learning about the principles and practice of yoga nidra. Through this book, discovering how to replace the pressure and tension of the stress response with refreshing energy will help you live a meaningful life that is healthy, happy, and fulfilling. However, simply knowing about it is not enough. The heart and soul of *Yoga Nidra for Complete Relaxation and Stress Relief* is in the experience of it. Find out for yourself! You will reap enormous benefits.

## Chapter 1

# The Seriousness of Stress and the Importance of Stress Relief

S tress. The very sound of the word is harsh, almost like nails being scraped down a chalkboard. Stressors are anything that causes stress. Can you identify with any of these stressors?

- You are being pulled in a million directions and you have too much to do with not enough time or money.

- Your job is getting on your last nerve. Your coworkers are hard to cope with, and you feel overworked and underpaid. However, you have to work to support yourself and those depending on you. There is no time to look for something else, even if there was something out there.

- Everywhere you look there is illness, divorce, financial trouble, addiction, and crime. Yikes!

Most of us are being bombarded by stress and its consequences including irritability, sleepless nights, exhaustion, sickness, aches and pains of all kinds, as well as lowered productivity, efficiency, and effectiveness. In other words, the heat is on.

Many of us would rather ignore stress than have to deal with it, hoping it will just go away. Others believe that stress is energizing and motivating and helps them keep going. Unfortunately, neither of these approaches will work for long.

Effective strategies and outlets are needed for handling modern-day stressors. *Yoga Nidra for Complete Relaxation and Stress Relief* is the way to go. This chapter will help you understand and personally assess your stress and its ramifications. Here is your opportunity to address the root causes of stress and tackle them on a fundamental level.

## What Is Stress?

Stress is a normal and instantaneous physiological reaction to pressure that is triggered by situational, physical, mental, or emotional tension. It does not matter if a threat is real or imagined. Stress can slowly creep up on us or can come on all of a sudden from out of the blue. It shows up in both obvious and subtle ways.

Stress occurs when a person perceives that the demand on them—ranging from minor irritations to major trauma—exceeds their personal coping abilities and their resources. Sometimes we deal with stress effectively while at other times we handle it poorly.

Stress is experienced whenever we feel threatened. For instance, being physically under attack by an opponent is clearly stressful, as are floods and fires. Just the same, going through life's adjustments, daily duties, and changes also has the potential for triggering unwanted stress, whether the changes are perceived as positive or negative. A few potential stressors include work-related pressures, family problems, financial issues, traffic jams, computer problems, waiting in line, and deadlines. Poor lifestyle choices such as inadequate nutrition, sleep deprivation, and addictions can make us more vulnerable to stress and add to its negative impact. Changes like getting a promotion, going on vacation, graduating, or getting married can also trigger stress.

Experiencing too much stress can cause unhappiness, sickness, poor relationships, anxiety, and lack of energy. If stress is not addressed appropriately and on a regular basis, it can lead to health issues that manifest physically, mentally, and/or emotionally.

Most folks who are often overwhelmed by stress either don't have a clue as to what to do about it or can't seem to find the time to handle stress appropriately. Others figure that living under constant pressure is normal and even helpful. Some people think they know enough about it or that stress doesn't matter very much. Few are aware of the ramifications of stress in their life, and most think that the way they react to stress is how others do too.

The truth is that typically, each person reacts differently to stressors. What is exhilarating and challenging to one person can drive someone else nuts. For example, a snowstorm is exciting and full of adventure for some people while others feel dread and worry upon even hearing a snowy weather forecast. Others ignore the snow completely. In another example, a computer glitch causes anxiety in some and feels like a challenging puzzle to others. These examples show how the same circumstance can create different reactions and responses in people.

Relaxation, in and of itself, is misunderstood and undervalued in our society. It is often associated with wasting time. It's considered unnecessary, even though relaxation is actually vital for health and happiness. Unfortunately, many assume they know how to relax: by relying on faulty behaviors like watching excessive TV, unnecessary or compulsive shopping, nonexistent to excessive exercise, tobacco use, and inappropriate eating and drinking.

## The Distraction Disadvantage and Its Causes

Most of us are out of practice when it comes to staying focused. This makes us easily distracted. We try to do too much in too short of time by racing through the to-do list. Our thoughts, actions, and feelings jump around as quickly as the flashing images and sounds of a televised thriller. It becomes really hard to stay focused with so much competing for our attention, which causes us to be increasingly more scattered. Attention span and memory are prone to shrink to almost nothing.

*Multitasking* seems smart but it does not work in the long run. Even though it seems like we are doing two or more things simultaneously, what really happens is that the brain rapidly switches back and forth from one task to another. While it can be useful in rote tasks that require little intelligent brainpower (walking while chewing gum), multitasking is detrimental in tasks requiring cognitive capacity. Multitasking actually changes brain matter itself (Loh and Kanai 2014). It contributes to stress, wastes time, lowers productivity, and hurts short- and long-term memory (Kuchinskas 2008). The brain is not capable of taking in and dealing with two different streams of information simultaneously. It is impossible for the brain to encode more than one stream of information fully into short-term memory at a time. Information will never make it into long-term memory if it does not go into short-term memory first. Either way, information cannot be recalled and put to use. This pattern contributes to forgetfulness, poor memory, and more stress (Merrill 2012).

*Connectivity creep* is another pattern invading practically everything. It starts with going online to look up something to complete a task. In no time at all, we are caught up in checking e-mail, scanning the news and social media sites, or gaming, making it hard to get back to the original intent of going online. Answering work e-mails and taking calls in the car and on weekends is the norm. Shortcuts and getting answers quickly seem more important than thinking something through carefully. Thoughtful problem solving and right action seem like a luxury of the past. Taking a break to enjoy a meal with a friend, having some family time, or enjoying the arts is often interrupted by this connectivity. Devices become vices. The stress reaction is continually firing and drains our energy, resources, and health down to nothing.

The *distraction disadvantage* refers to multitasking, connectivity creep, and similar behaviors. At first, these distraction patterns seem harmless enough until they carry over into daily life. Being mentally distracted can lead to a stressful chain reaction. For instance, stress quickly increases when one feels under pressure to get somewhere on time, especially when having to frantically search for lost keys that were mindlessly tossed somewhere while multitasking. Composure is lost and tempers flare. In another example, accidents and injuries are more likely to happen when preoccupied.

Stress is triggered when boundaries between personal time and work life are blurred. It seems impossible to get blocks of time to do any thinking or get anything done anymore because of multitasking and all the disruptions that come from the continual connectivity at work, home, and in the car. Have you ever looked back on your day and asked, "I was busy running around all day, but what did I get done?" No matter what causes stress, all of us experience the same stress reaction.

## The Stress Reaction

The *stress reaction* refers to the fight-flight-freeze response. It is activated every time stress is experienced for survival and to protect us from threats. The *fight-or-flight response* was identified by W. B. Cannon in the 1920s and further clarified by Hans Selye, an endocrinologist. More recently, the *freeze response* was described in *The Body Bears the Burden* (2014), by Robert Scaer, MD, and in *Waking the Tiger* (1997), by Peter Levine, PhD, among others.

The brain constantly processes what is being observed in the environment by collecting information from what it senses through what is being thought, seen, heard, felt, and smelled. This is extremely important for survival, especially in humanity's early days of being threatened by wild animals or warring clans. When real or imagined stress is detected, the *autonomic nervous system* (ANS) and the *endocrine system* both get involved in responding. The endocrine system is composed of all the different glands that produce and secrete hormones that regulate the activity of cells and organs. Under stress, the part of the limbic brain called the *amygdala* instantly evaluates the degree of threat and immediately triggers a cascade of hormonal reactions in the body in preparation for either fighting, fleeing, or freezing. Our rational, thinking mind is automatically left out of this equation since immediate survival is of uppermost priority. After all, it might be too late if we had to take time to think through an impending crisis. Instead, the amygdala picks the best survival reaction for us and instantly goes to work.

Even though most of us are not in danger of physical threats most of the time, the stress reaction is still regularly activated in all its glory. This occurs whether a threat is real or imagined. Our thoughts and beliefs can quickly trigger the stress response. For instance, feeling afraid of getting chewed out by the boss will just as quickly trigger the stress response and can be even harder on you than the real thing. Even though we may be physically prepared to punch his or her lights out or to escape, it is not appropriate to do so. Instead, we typically grin and bear it. This leaves the body all revved up and ready for action, as if a tiger is breathing down your neck instead of your boss. You might notice yourself saying something like, "I could have wrung his neck" (fight response) or "I couldn't wait to get out of there" (flight response). While this acknowledges stress, it does not come close to solving much of anything. This pent-up energy will brew and fester if it is not effectively released in a timely manner.

Unfortunately, the fight-flight-freeze reaction can become the constant state of affairs in your body. This happens when you're being continually inundated by stressors—big or little—and when you do not have the necessary time and tools needed to recover and return to a balanced state. When the stress reaction stays in high gear, it takes its toll. This dysregulation can damage the heart, contribute to chronic muscle tension, disrupt digestion and elimination, trigger problems associated with inflammation, and can contribute to mental and emotional distress (Collingwood 2007; APA 2014; Mayo Clinic 2013).

To handle stress better, it is important to have an understanding of the fight-flight-freeze reaction and its implications. The best place to start is by learning a little more about the autonomic nervous system and the endocrine system. Following that, we will take a close look at the relaxation response.

## The Autonomic Nervous System

The ANS is always operating in an effort to maintain internal functions normally. It is part of the peripheral nervous system and is composed of a network of nerve fibers that extends throughout the body, connecting the brain with various organs such as the heart, stomach, and intestines. Some muscles are also controlled by the ANS. All this operates involuntarily and reflexively. It controls things like breathing, blood pressure variations, digestive track secretions, and whether our eyes are dilating or constricting. As we shall see, the fine balance needed for good health is disrupted by ongoing stress and can cause serious problems.

The two main branches of the ANS are the sympathetic and the parasympathetic nervous systems. Both systems are supposed to work together to maintain balance and harmony internally, whether we are being hit with stress or not. To help remember which is which, think of the sympathetic nervous system as *sympathizing* with us when we are stressed out.

## The Sympathetic Nervous System and the Stress Reaction

The sympathetic branch of the nervous system activates the fight-flight-freeze reaction and gears up whenever stress and threats are detected. Happening in a fraction of a second, it enables you to fight harder, run more quickly, see more clearly, and breathe better than you normally would for self-protection. This happens whether it is appropriate or feasible to fight, run, or freeze. The amount of threat—or whether the danger is real or imagined—does not matter.

When appropriate, the fight-or-flight part of the reaction is a real lifesaver if you are in a dangerous neighborhood, violent home, or in a war zone with the need to get away fast or fight dearly for your life. And sometimes, it is safer to freeze and stay put rather than to fight or run.

### Fight-or-Flight Reaction

Here are the key reactions that instantaneously occur on a reflexive, unconscious, and involuntary basis when there is a real or perceived threat, large or small:

- The hormone *adrenaline* (sometimes called epinephrine) increases heart rate, elevates blood pressure, and boosts energy supplies.

- Breathing increases to deliver more oxygen to the major muscles, especially the legs for running.

■ Muscular tension increases.

■ Pupils dilate to improve vision.

■ Another hormone, *norepinephrine*, increases sensory awareness and heightens responsiveness and focus for better problem solving (being hyperalert).

■ Blood vessels in the skin constrict to limit bleeding while diverting energy to more important areas. This constriction is "hair-raising" and can cause goose bumps where hair is absent. The skin gets clammy and becomes pale (and might result in cold hands, sweaty palms, and/or perspiration).

■ Hormonal levels change in males (testosterone) and in females (oxytocin).

■ To be ready for injury, a steroid hormone called *cortisol* is released that dulls pain. It also gears up the immune system to deliver infection-fighting white blood cells whenever and wherever needed. The immune system first increases, but if the stress is prolonged or too much cortisol is in the system, immunity is suppressed in order to divert energy back to the heart and lungs.

■ Cortisol starts conserving energy by curtailing functions that are not essential for bodily functions or would interfere with the fight-flight-freeze response.

■ Digestion, kidney functions, and tissue repair are slowed to divert energy to where it is needed.

■ Decreased salivation levels occur (dry mouth is common).

■ The reproductive system and growth processes are suppressed.

**Freeze Reaction**

When the fight-or-flight reaction is not possible and not an option due to the threat involved, the ANS automatically changes from the fight-or-flight reaction into the freeze response. Like the fight-or-flight response, freezing is a subconscious reaction that happens involuntarily when the brain's limbic system determines that staying still is the optimal strategy for survival. This is likely to happen due to an extreme threat or the circumstances involved. An example is "the deer in the headlights" reaction when an animal automatically stops "dead in its tracks" until the predator is gone.

Have you ever been "frozen with fear" or at a loss for words and unable to speak when under pressure? Have you ever felt "scared stiff" and shut down physically or emotionally? You were probably holding your breath or breathing shallowly, signaling a form of the freeze response. Once again, these immobilizing reactions can happen whether the stressor is actual or imagined. The freeze reaction has a few results:

- Feelings of being helpless, hopeless, numb, dissociated, walled off, powerless, and lifeless become present.

- *Endorphins* are secreted that reduce panic in order to increase chances of survival and numb pain in the event of an attack (or death).

- Immobilization, which is temporarily paralyzing, occurs.

Recovery from the freeze response typically starts with shaking, followed by the fight-or-flight response to enable the animal or person to get away or fight if needed. This important process is necessary to discharge the effects of the stress reaction and reduce the likelihood of long-lasting effects, like traumatic stress.

## Lucy's Story

Let's look at an example of the fight-flight-freeze response that happened while writing this book. On a beautiful spring day, my husband, Dave, let our lap dog, Lucy, out into our backyard. He noticed that her rawhide bone was in the yard, so he went over to pick it up. When she took off running, he assumed that she wanted to play catch. Wrong! She had spotted a mother raccoon and her two babies. Instantly, she started barking and chasing them (fight response). She has never run so fast! All three raccoons took off running (flight response) to save their hides. The mother raccoon ran under the house, and the babies scattered in two different directions. In its haste, one baby fell into a window well and was trapped. It was fighting for its life by screaming at the top of its lungs and trying its hardest to climb to safety. The whole neighborhood must have heard the racket. Unfortunately, Lucy grabbed the other baby and ran off. Meanwhile, Dave was yelling at the dog to stop and for me to come help. His heart was pumping and he was sweating bullets. I was stunned when I got outside and saw what was happening; I briefly froze in my tracks until I could get my bearings (freeze response). Dave finally got the raccoon away from Lucy and was holding it by the tail. We saw that it was injured and needed help. We remembered that we had a have-a-heart cage, so I ran to get it. In no time at all, that raccoon was inside it. Whew! What a relief. Now, what about the other baby? By this time, it was no longer screaming, so we thought it had gotten itself out of the window well. Wrong again! It was lying down perfectly still and hiding under the leaves. Overwhelmed, it could no longer fight or flee, so it froze, becoming invisible so it wouldn't be bothered. We would have overlooked it if we hadn't searched carefully. I ran to get Dave some gloves so he could reach in and get it out. He grabbed it by the tail and returned it to safety.

As we shall soon find out, the rate of recovery after stress becomes important for all of us experiencing the flight-fight-freeze response during stressful episodes.

### Tend-and-Befriend Response

The tend-and-befriend response, identified by Shelley E. Taylor, PhD, and her colleagues in 2000, is thought to be a variation of the freeze response. It's mostly found in females due to the measurable release of the hormone *oxytocin* for improving survival rates in themselves and their offspring. It refers to the tendency not to take the risk of getting hurt by fighting or fleeing but to stay put to start tending and watching over others, like when there are kids and home at stake. It is also characterized by grouping together for protection and support, and to diffuse the stressful situation. Furthermore, stress is released by talking and collaborating.

Doing this research shed some new light on my first childhood music recital, which I dreaded. When it was my turn, I sat there stiff as a board. I could not think, I could not move, and then I started shaking. Looking back, my nervous system was actually trying to protect me. During this situation, I could not escape (flight), nor could I scream out in fear (fight). The only option left was to freeze. I felt like a stupid failure afterward and was scared of recitals for years. My self-esteem plummeted. It would have been really helpful to talk with someone about what had happened (tend-and-befriend). After being calmed down and comforted, it would have been a relief to be reassured that what happened was a normal reaction to stress and not my inadequacy as a person or as a musician. Freezing was an automatic and unconscious response, and there was nothing I could have done differently at the time. Shaking was my system's way of naturally discharging the stress hormones. Freezing up has happened to me during other testing situations and before speaking in front of others, even though I knew the material and was prepared. First, my heart would start pounding, my hands would get cold and clammy, and my stomach would knot up (fight-or-flight response). Then my mind would go blank and I would start shaking (freeze response). Now I know to use relaxation training as part of my preparation, to use relaxation skills to turn the stress response off under pressure, and to talk about it afterward (tend-and-befriend). Can you relate to my experience?

### The Parasympathetic Nervous System and the Relaxation Response

The *parasympathetic nervous system* is the second branch of the ANS. It functions by signaling to the body that the stress is over, and it initiates the relaxation response. Hormone levels are returned to normal once a perceived threat has passed. As adrenaline and cortisol levels drop, heart rate and blood pressure return to baseline levels, and other systems resume their regular activities.

The *relaxation response* was identified in the 1960s by Herbert Benson, MD, a scientist at Harvard Medical School and the director of the Behavioral Medicine Division at Beth Israel Deaconess Medical Center in Boston. The relaxation response is accountable for many things:

- Turns the stress response off

- Reduces the stress hormones (adrenaline, norepinephrine, cortisol)

- Regulates the heart rate and pulse to healthy levels

- Lowers high blood pressure

- Slows the respiratory rate and decreases oxygen consumption

- Decreases muscle tension

- Increases blood flow to major muscles

- Reduces fatigue and increases energy

- Changes genetic activities that are in opposition to those associated with stress

The changes listed above can result in these benefits:

- Digestion naturally occurs

- Breathing becomes regular

- A sense of calmness is produced

- Brain functions increase for improved attention and decision-making

- Aging process slows down

- Less effort is required

- Anxiety is decreased

- Sleep improves

- Happiness, satisfaction, and the ability to focus increase

## How the Natural Stress Reaction Gets Offtrack

The body's stress reaction system was not designed for managing chronic stress. It was meant to handle acute, short-term stress on an as-needed basis for protection and survival. For better or worse, dangerous threats to us were usually over with quickly, and equilibrium was reestablished.

These days, physical attacks are relatively uncommon. The American Psychological Association has identified the top causes of stress in its 2013 national survey on the subject. They are:

1. *Job pressure:* Coworker tension, bosses, work overload

2. *Money:* Loss of a job, reduced retirement, medical expenses

3. *Health:* Health crisis or terminal or chronic illness

4. *Relationships:* Divorce, death of spouse, arguments with friends, loneliness

5. *Poor nutrition:* Inadequate nutrition, caffeine, processed foods, refined sugars

6. *Media overload:* Television, radio, Internet, e-mail, social networking

7. *Sleep deprivation:* Inability to release the stress hormones (adrenaline, norepinephrine, cortisol) interfering with the ability to sleep (APA 2013)

Obviously, these stressors are quite different from being in danger of physical harm. Modern-day stressors are continual and can keep the stress response in high gear. The constant state of stressful overstimulation can take over and make it more and more difficult to recover from stress and all its ramifications. Imagine that there is a stress reaction faucet that continuously floods your system. First, the parasympathetic nervous system and the relaxation response get rusty. Over time, the stress reaction can get frozen in the "on" position and the automatic and much-needed transition from the stress response to the relaxation response fails. Staying constantly revved up makes it very difficult to recover one's equilibrium, have good health, and be able to really relax and enjoy living life to the fullest.

If the nervous system does not have an outlet to release the stress reaction or becomes overwhelmed by too many hassles (big or small), it becomes deregulated and cannot do its job correctly. Instead of returning to balance, digestion, tissue repair, and the immune system stay suppressed, and the heart rate stays elevated longer than needed. It may get harder and harder to fall asleep or stay asleep during the night. Overexposure to the stress reaction increases the risk and severity of numerous health problems, including muscular tension (headaches, backaches, stomachaches, and so on), and contributes to stress-related disorders like high blood pressure (hypertension), constipation, diarrhea, diabetes, infertility, and chronic fatigue syndrome (APA 2013). It can also have a negative impact on the brain itself, causing certain important parts of it to change (Krugers, Hoogenraad, and Groc 2010).

Physical and psychological stress can influence us to "reward ourselves" to help us feel better temporarily. Have you ever reached for something "bad" to calm yourself down after being stressed? If this becomes a habit, it can lead to making poor lifestyle choices such as chronic unhealthy eating habits, inadequate sleep, excessive drinking, inappropriate drug use, and/or tobacco use. Resorting to behaviors such as these is like throwing gasoline on a fire—these actions flare up into a host of medical problems as well as other personal and social troubles. Shawn Talbot, PhD, reports in his book, *The Cortisol Connection: Why Stress Makes You Fat and Ruins Your Health—And What You Can Do About It* (2011), that caffeine, sleep deprivation, and alcohol all increase cortisol, the stress hormone. Excessive cortisol has been shown to play a role in a host of chronic diseases. It depresses the immune system, elevates blood pressure and blood glucose (sugar), increases inflammation, lowers sex drive, produces acne, decreases bone density, and contributes to weight gain, especially abdominal fat. Yuck!

Fortunately, there are tools at our disposal to remedy this dangerous situation. We can each take positive action to prevent and/or cope with stress. We can use the relaxation techniques that are found in this book to get ourselves back on track and into balance. With regular practice, we can bring the sympathetic and parasympathetic systems back into their proper relationship and enjoy a happy and healthy life!

## Identifying Your Sources of Stress

The causes of stress are either controllable or uncontrollable. The trick is to learn *how to control the controllable* and figure out *how to cope with the uncontrollable*. Living and working under constant pressure can lull you into the false belief that the symptoms of stress are normal. We start ignoring muscular tension—and then wonder why our head hurts. We may start assuming that poor digestion is normal. We convince ourselves that everyone suffers from insomnia. Some even believe these symptoms are a badge of honor and courage, symbolizing their hard work and dedication. Not so. This is dangerous and can lead to a whole host of problems.

A first step in managing stress is to assess your sources and levels of stress. Stress is an individual matter for everyone. It can stem from environmental, psychological, or physical sources. What sends one person over the edge may be regarded as a challenge that motivates someone else. No matter what triggers the stress reaction in you, the important thing is to recognize it and break the cycle.

# Assess Your Stress Questionnaire

How you react to stress is very personal. This assessment reviews how stress manifests itself physically, energetically, mentally, and emotionally. Each of these aspects of ourselves is referred to as a *kosha* (pronounced *KOH-shah*) in the yogic system and is explained in chapter 2.

For now, check off the situations and typical symptoms that you generally experience. We will come back to and work with this assessment to support and guide your practice of yoga nidra by identifying the qualities and characteristics that counterbalance the symptoms of stress. Use a notebook or journal for jotting down your answers, adding your other personal stressors, and for notes on your progress.

## Situational and Environmental Stressors

Situational and environmental stress comes from reactions to outside sources in the shape of people, places, circumstances, and events. Review the following list and mark the ones that typically bother you.

_____ Exposure to dangerous neighborhoods, abusive homes, and/or war zones

_____ Deadlines

_____ Traffic jams, parking problems

_____ Too much to do, too little time

_____ Waiting

_____ Running late

_____ Financial problems

_____ Health-related problems (health crisis, illness)

_____ Media overload (Internet, social media, e-mails, texts, TV, radio)

_____ Equipment breakdowns

_____ Loud or distracting noises that startle you or get on your nerves

_____ Losing things

_____ Weather-related problems

_____ Local and world news, politics

_____ Unsatisfying work

_____ Unemployment or underemployment

_____ Life changes and adjustments (marriage, divorce, birth, graduation, retirement, death of a loved one, et cetera)

_____ Problems with family, friends, or coworkers (poor communication, disagreements, et cetera)

_____ Caring for children, parents, or a sick family member or friend

_____ Everyday responsibilities (paying bills, home and car maintenance, chores)

_____ Other

## Physical Symptoms (Anna Maya Kosha)

One of the major symptoms of stress is physical. Yogis refer to the physical system in Sanskrit as the _anna maya kosha_ (pronounced AH-nah MY-ah KOH-shah). Physical problems are distracting, uncomfortable, and time consuming. Check off your common physical reactions and results of stressful living. As a reminder, it is important to rule out medical problems by having age-appropriate health checkups and to see your health care provider when necessary.

_____ Tension headaches

_____ Sweaty palms

_____ Sleep problems (too much or too little sleep, inability to get to sleep or stay asleep)

_____ Fatigue, lethargy

_____ Clumsiness, being accident-prone

_____ Back pain

_____ Stomachaches, indigestion

_____ Diarrhea or constipation

_____ Skin rashes

_____ Frequent blushing

_____ Dry mouth

_____ Muscle tension

_____ Cold hands or feet

_____ Grinding teeth, jaw tension

_____ Nutritional problems (inadequate nutrition, eating too much or too little)

_____ Substance abuse (alcohol, tobacco, and prescription or illegal drugs)

_____ Feeling ill at ease

_____ Feeling ungrounded, uprooted, or disconnected

_____ Numbness

_____ Feeling empty

_____ Other

## Energy Body Symptoms (Prana Maya Kosha)

Our energetic life force is also affected by stress. Yogis refer to this system as the *prana maya kosha* (pronounced PRAH-nah MY-ah KOH-shah). This can be monitored and measured primarily by the rate, rhythm, and quality of the breath, as well as your energy level.

_____ Shallow breathing

_____ Arrhythmic, uneven breathing

_____ Upper chest instead of abdominal breathing

_____ Fast breathing (twelve to sixteen breaths per minute is average for adults at rest)

_____ Holding your breath

_____ Sighing

_____ Inhalations longer than the exhalations

_____ Mouth breathing (unless physically necessary)

_____ Either the right or left nostril dominates breathing

_____ One or both nostrils are typically blocked

_____ Feeling tired often

_____ Feeling hyper or restless often

_____ Other

## Psychological Symptoms (Mano Maya Kosha)

Stress is also psychological in nature and can show up emotionally and mentally as a cause and an outcome of stress. This system is referred to as the *mano maya kosha* (pronounced MAH-no MY-ah KOH-shah) by yogis. Anger, impatience, depression, and guilt are typical examples from the emotional arena. Worry, lack of concentration, and making mistakes are characteristic of how stress manifests mentally.

Check off your typical emotional symptoms:

_____ Feeling edgy, nervous, or uneasy

_____ Depression

_____ Crying frequently or unexpectedly

_____ Feeling pressure

_____ Anger

_____ Apathy

_____ Dissatisfaction

_____ Tension

_____ Fear

_____ Embarrassment

_____ Guilt

_____ Sadness

_____ Losing your temper

_____ Withdrawing from others

_____ Being argumentative, critical, or bossy

_____ Other

Check off your typical mental symptoms:

_____ Confusion

_____ Forgetfulness or memory loss, foggy thinking

_____ Constant worry

_____ Boredom

_____ Indecision

_____ Irrational thoughts

_____ Making too many mistakes or errors

_____ Unwanted thoughts

_____ Decrease in attention span

_____ Feeling scattered

_____ Obsessing

_____ Easily distractible

_____ Other

## Belief Symptoms (Vijnana Maya Kosha)

Faulty or limiting beliefs we have about ourselves can run us dry and ragged. Yogis refer to this system as the *vijnana maya kosha* (pronounced *veej-NAH-nah MY-ah KOH-shah*). The beliefs below are associated with the chakra system of health and well-being (see chapter 5 for more on the chakras). Check off your typical thoughts and beliefs:

_____ I am not enough/I feel unworthy.

_____ I often feel unsafe.

_____ I often deny or ignore my needs.

_____ I often feel numb, dull, or unsure of my emotions.

_____ I hold a lot of regrets and guilt.

_____ I have a poor opinion of myself.

_____ I often feel shame.

_____ I believe I am unlovable.

_____ I carry a lot of grief.

_____ It's hard for me to forgive.

_____ It's hard to express myself truthfully or kindly.

_____ It's hard for me to see the big picture.

_____ I rarely use or trust my intuition.

_____ I don't think I am smart enough.

_____ I hold on and have attachments.

_____ I feel unconnected spiritually.

_____ Other

## Analyze Your Stressors and Symptoms

Now that you have identified your main stressors and symptoms, take time to look at them carefully to help you know where to concentrate your efforts for the biggest impact on gaining stress relief. Focus your attention on the categories that have five or more items checked off. These areas indicate the types of stress that are pervasive in your life, whether you realize it or not. Pull out your journal and answer these important follow-up questions to better understand your unique stress situation:

1. What categories are predominant for you? List them.

2. Did you notice any surprises? What are they?

3. Are there trends? Name them.

4. What self-care measures can you undertake?

5. Is it time for outside help? If yes, please elaborate.

# How to Limit Stress and Activate the Relaxation Response

Just because we need and want to relax doesn't make it easy. Relaxation techniques are needed that will stop the inappropriate activity of the sympathetic nervous system and break the train of stressful thoughts. Since the stress response is subconscious and automatic, we must learn ways to intervene as well as use skills to break the cycle of stress. Even though diversion and entertainment has its place, activities like simply sitting still, hobbies, reading the news, or watching television are not enough to produce the physiological changes needed to activate the relaxation response, according to Herbert Benson, MD, co-author of *The Relaxation Revolution* (2010).

Yoga nidra purposely and deliberately activates the parasympathetic nervous system and brings the relaxation response to life, providing quick and reliable relief. It focuses on effective strategies that include specialized breathing techniques, relaxation training, visualization, and meditation. Reactions to stress and our recovery time improve the more these skills are practiced.

So if you are feeling bad that you checked off way more items on the Assess Your Stress questionnaire than you thought possible, and you're feeling even more stressed out than before, there's still good news. In fact, there's great news: you can begin to relieve your stress and relax *right now*. All you need is your breath. And after a minute or two (the more the better, though), I promise you will feel less tension. I invite you to read on.

## Diaphragmatic Breathing

Stress relief does not have to be complicated or time-consuming. In fact, it is as simple as practicing some yogic breathing. *Diaphragmatic breathing (dirgha pranayama)* is a simple, straightforward way to turn off the stress response and turn on the relaxation response.

As we know, it is impossible to consciously tell our heart to slow down or make our palms quit sweating, since those functions are not under our conscious control. Even though breathing is automatic too, we *can* consciously control it. While stressing out, breathing automatically becomes fast, shallow, and arrhythmic. Intentionally changing our breathing pattern to diaphragmatic breathing causes the air to go deeply into the lungs rather than staying shallow. Doing so physiologically connects us directly to our sympathetic and parasympathetic nervous systems and provides stress relief via the relaxation response.

In addition, the rhythm and rate of your breathing makes a difference. Under stress, the inhalation gets longer and the exhalation shortens. This negatively impacts heart rate, blood pressure, and can trigger panicky feelings. Learn to reverse this pattern and feel relaxed energy quickly with the following breathing exercise. Get in the habit of breathing diaphragmatically throughout the day, whether you are feeling stressed or not.

## Diaphragmatic Breathing Exercise

Begin by noticing how you are breathing right now. Notice if you are breathing through your mouth or nose. Without changing it, become aware of its pace by noticing if it seems fast or slow to you. Where are you feeling your breath? Is it most noticeable at your nostrils, or can you feel it in your throat, chest, or abdomen?

Start breathing through your nose so that your inhalation and your exhalation are in balance. This means that if you are breathing in for a count of four, breathe out for a count of four.

Once familiarized and comfortable with this, begin to extend your exhalation so it becomes longer. In other words, if you are breathing in for a count of four, begin to breathe out for a count of five to ten.

Breathe this way for at least one to two minutes, or until the tension has decreased and your energy improves.

Refer to appendix 2 for detailed instructions on this and other specialized breathing techniques. Additional yogic breathing techniques are included in each of the three yoga nidra practices as well as in appendix 3.

## Anne's Story

Last week, Anne was getting ready to go to the airport to catch a flight. Before she even left the house, the airlines informed her of flight delays. She was assured that she would make her connections. At the airport, however, it became obvious that more delays were in store, and her connections were shot. Instead of stressing out, she remembered that she could stay calm and keep her wits by focusing on her breathing. Anne made sure she was breathing a long, deep, and slow exhalation followed by a full inhalation. This kept the stress response in check. She also knew that staying in the moment, rather than letting her mind race into worrying about future problems, would be smart. After all, she reminded herself, she would eventually reach her destination. So rather than getting upset, she was able to feel like she was in a center of calm amid the chaos that people were experiencing around her. Arguing with the airline representatives (fight response) would not help matters. It could cause undue worry, get her heart racing, increase her blood pressure, and make her feel lousy. Anne felt so thankful that she had practiced breathing this way through yoga nidra.

## Resiliency to Stress

There are people who are more resilient to and can recover from the stress response and get back to normal sooner while others take longer. *Resiliency* is the ability to withstand stress, rise above it, and bounce back stronger than ever.

Let's revisit the story of my dog and the raccoons to better understand resiliency and recovery. Lucy forgot about the raccoon right away. The next time she went out in the yard, she acted as if raccoons didn't exist. My husband started working off his stress physically by going out into the garden and pulling weeds, and I started telling my friends what had happened and wrote about it in my journal. Later, we went for a walk and talked about what had happened. In fact, we continued to talk on and off all day. Walking helped to release the stress hormones that had built up, and talking helped us process what had happened to get it out of our systems. If we hadn't used some form of release to help us recover, the day's stressful event would have continued to affect us physically, causing our hearts to continue racing, among other side effects. Likewise, it would have been harmful if we had started to continually worry about Lucy hurting or getting hurt by a raccoon every time she went outside. Instead, we blocked off the place where the raccoons were living to prevent future problems.

Even though some of us are more resilient than others, there is a lot that can be practiced to adapt to stress without lasting effects. We can learn to "roll with the punches" as well as to use stressors for motivation and inspiration to make positive changes.

Some of the best ways to develop better resiliency can be found right in the center of the philosophy, principles, and practices of yoga nidra. These qualities include cultivating self-awareness, practicing acceptance, having a positive attitude, developing a spiritual side, and having the ability to clear your mind and calm restlessness through guided relaxation, breathing techniques, and meditation.

## What to Remember

- In our busy world, feeling stress is a common part of life and living. It is here to stay. Therefore, learning and practicing real relaxation is no longer optional.

- The stress response (fight-flight-freeze or tend-befriend reaction) occurs whenever stress is experienced as a result of the sympathetic nervous system. This automatic reaction is not meant for handling chronic but acute stress, and it occurs for actual and imaginary threats.

- The parasympathetic nervous system (hopefully) counteracts the stress reaction with the relaxation response.

- The distraction disadvantage, including multitasking and connectivity creep, increases stress and leads to poor memory, a short attention span, and mistakes. Counteract it by trying to complete tasks from start to finish. Stay focused and handle one thing at a time. Then, watch your ability to remember things grow and your concentration increase. Enjoyment will expand as your ability to stay present develops, enabling you to truly enjoy a beautiful sunrise without searching for a camera, or really savor the flavor and texture of delicious food. Taking time to listen to others without the distraction of formulating what you are going to say will improve relationships and give you space to respond from your intuitive heart.

- It is vitally important to get a grip on stress, practice relaxation skills, and be more resilient in order to have the health and energy to live a happier and meaningful life.

- Yoga nidra is a valuable technique that gives you the skills needed to experience conscious deep relaxation. It will help you understand and overcome physical, mental, and emotional stress.

- Lean toward peace.

## Chapter 2

# Understanding Yoga Nidra

Yoga is perhaps the world's original answer to stress relief. In ancient times, yogis were primarily interested in exploring the human capacity for consciousness and enlightenment. Some dedicated practitioners of yoga may achieve enlightenment, but most people today are content with the many benefits of the practices because they lead to healthier bodies, calmer and clearer mental and emotional states, and less stressful daily lives.

The word "yoga" means "union" or "joining." This union refers to the joining of different aspects of ourselves so that we do not feel scattered or isolated, get stressed, and become sick. It brings about the natural integration of our body, mind, and spirit. Yoga refers to the joining and balancing of our light and dark places, the concrete and the abstract, the internal and external, and our masculine and feminine aspects. It especially refers to the union of our individual self with our higher, divine Self, and the oneness of all. It is neither a religion nor sport. Yoga is really about becoming whole and balanced. Fortunately, it also gives us practical tools for doing so.

Over thousands of years, the practices of hatha yoga, yoga nidra, meditation, and other methods were developed to accomplish this. Hatha yoga focuses on the physical aspect of yoga and includes the practice of physical postures (*asana*), breathing techniques (*pranayama*), and directing sensory awareness from an external to an internal perspective (*pratyahara*). Meditation (*dharana, dhyana,* and *samadhi*) focuses on mental attitude and awareness, affecting not only the mind but also the body, emotions, and spirit. Yoga nidra, both a pratyahara technique to draw the senses inward and a particular state of conscious awareness, is positioned right in the center of hatha yoga and meditation.

## Yoga Nidra: Experience and Benefits

Yoga nidra is a powerful and unique state of awareness in which the body profoundly relaxes, the thinking mind fades away, emotions seem to evaporate, alertness magnifies, and awareness becomes crisp and clear.

It begins with a very deep state of relaxation occurring physically, energetically, mentally, and emotionally. It serves as a natural prelude to meditation. As this happens, we experience a level of consciousness that precedes all awareness. Not only is it stress-free, it is extremely healing, restorative, and powerful.

What is experienced is awareness without words, thoughts, images, feelings, and other sensations. This awareness connects us with where our innate wisdom, intelligence, and intuition naturally exist. Pure bliss. Yoga nidra is a delightful route to the heart and soul of yoga—and yourself.

It is done lying down in the relaxation pose (*shavasana*, pronounced *shah-VAH-sah-nah*) and powerfully combines specialized breathing techniques (pranayama), sensory training and control (pratyahara), and meditation (dharana, dhyana, and samadhi). This progression naturally leads us into conscious deep relaxation, the experience of meditative awareness, and experiencing our true Self (Atma).

Through all my years of personal practice, study, and teaching others, I have not found a more effective or reliable method for relieving stress, feeling the peacefulness of relaxation, healing and restoring the body, understanding and managing emotions, quieting the mind, experiencing unbounded consciousness, and awakening the compassionate heart than yoga nidra.

Yoga nidra is a wonderful and natural complement to the healing and life-enriching benefits of practicing yoga postures and specialized breathing. In fact, a hatha yoga practice is never complete—and would be like a one-winged bird—without time devoted to being in shavasana at the end of a session. On the other hand, yoga nidra can certainly be practiced on its own without practicing yoga postures.

Here are a few things yoga nidra can do:

- Activate the relaxation response and deactivate the stress response (which improves functioning of the sympathetic and parasympathetic nervous systems and the endocrine system).

- Increase immunity and the ability to fight germs and infections (Kumar 2013a, 82–94)

- Improve heart functioning by lowering blood pressure and cholesterol (Pandya and Kumar 2007)

- Decrease pain

- Improve control of fluctuating blood glucose and symptoms associated with diabetes (Amita et al. 2009)

- Significantly improve anxiety, depression, and well-being in patients with menstrual irregularities and in those having psychological problems (Rani et al. 2011)

- Manage pre- and postsurgical conditions (Kumar 2013a, 56)

- Reduce insomnia and improve sleep: while not intended as a substitute for sleep, one hour of effective yoga nidra practice is equivalent to about four hours of sleep (Kumar 2013a)

- Increase energy, especially when needed most

- Reduce worry and enhance clear thinking and problem solving

- Improve and refresh your outlook

- Replace mood swings and emotional upsets with greater emotional understanding and stability

- Develop intuition and increase creativity

- Improve meditation and enhance its benefits

- Integrate, heal, and revitalize your body, mind, and spirit

- Enhance your Self-awareness and ability to experience *witness consciousness* (defined later in this chapter)

- Transform thoughts and feelings of separation into a direct experience of wholeness

Finally, one of yoga nidra's prime benefits is that it brings yoga's essential teachings to life that have been handed down to us over the ages from the Upanishads, *Yoga Sutras* of Patanjali, Bhagavad Gita, Tantric texts, and others.

## Yoga's Essential Teachings

Yoga philosophers have given us new levels of understanding regarding the causes of stress and how to relieve it. This is a synthesis that draws from different Yoga philosophies.

It is believed that our true Self and the essential core of our being is eternally peaceful, luminous, joyful, loving, and compassionate. Furthermore, it is all knowing, indescribable, unwavering, indestructible, unblemished, ageless, and wise. Some Yoga masters call this core *purusha* and others call it the *Atman* (universal soul) or *Atma* (individual soul). Instead of using purusha, we will use Atma, Atman, or Self in this book. "Atman" is translated as the "transcendental Self" in Georg Feuerstein's *The Shambhala Encyclopedia of Yoga*. He states, "The Self (Atman, purusha) is one's authentic identity apart from all one's roles and is deemed immortal and immutable" (1997, 265). Yoga nidra enables us to experience the Atma firsthand.

43

The concept of Atman does not have an exact English equivalent, but "Self" comes closest. Similar concepts can be found in other philosophical traditions and go by many names including the "spiritual Self," "pure Spirit," "essential Self," and "True Nature." Christians call it the "soul" and "the kingdom of heaven." Buddhists and Hindus generally refer to it as "pure awareness."

Patanjali, an ancient Classical Yoga master and the recognized author of the *Yoga Sutras* (200 BCE), provides us with the needed foundations and the necessary instructions to facilitate our understanding of this. Patanjali's Yoga Sutra I.2 and I.3 say, "Yoga is the settling of the mind into silence. When the mind is settled, we are established in our essential nature, which is unbounded consciousness. Our essential nature is usually overshadowed by the activity of the mind" (Shearer 1982, 90). Nischala Joy Devi interprets this sutra from Sanskrit to English as: "Yoga is the uniting of consciousness in the heart. United in the heart, consciousness is steadied, then we abide in our true nature— joy. At other times, we identify with the rays of consciousness which fluctuate and encourage our perceived suffering" (Devi 2007, 280). Instead of identifying with our true Self, Yoga Sutras I.4, I.5, and I.6 say that we typically identify with five mental activities that may or may not cause problems: understanding, misunderstanding, imagination, sleep, and memory.

The stilling of the mind and the awakening of the compassionate heart is a fundamental and central goal of Yoga. Realizing this point of view helps us extinguish the root causes of much of our stress. We still remain fully engaged in living, including all its ups and downs, but with moment-to-moment awareness, mental clarity, emotional stability, and intuitive wisdom. Even when stressful things are challenging us and need our attention, there is a deep reservoir of inner peace inside that is based on a solid, joyful foundation rather than one built on stress. Persistent practice, patience, detachment, and time are needed to develop this understanding. Yoga nidra gives us the practical means for quieting mental ruckus and opening our heart for this to happen.

## Yoga Values and Fosters Freedom

Sutra I.13 of the ancient *Yoga Sutras of Patanjali* focuses on finding freedom from stress and suffering and gaining peace of mind. Practicing postures, as beneficial as they are, is not emphasized. It says, "The practice of yoga is the commitment to become established in the state of freedom," as interpreted by Alistair Shearer (1982, 92). Nischala Joy Devi translates this verse as "Devoted practice, *Abhyasa*, cultivates the unfolding of consciousness" (2007, 280).

Yoga helps us foster freedom by showing us how to form an easier relationship and connection with our outer and inner worlds. Yoga nidra is a valuable tool for knowing this freedom. It provides us with a path for coming home to our essential, unbounded Self.

In the outer world, our external efforts and material possessions have a definite purpose and a place. However, they will not yield lasting happiness due to the changing nature of things, thoughts, circumstances, relationships, feelings, emotions, and the like. When we have the capacity to impartially witness and watch these things change, we no longer identify with them so strongly. This is replaced with a new and larger identity—that of our essential Self. We have the opportunity to practice this during yoga nidra.

## The Importance of Witness Consciousness

It is valuable to have an understanding of *witness consciousness* and *pure consciousness* before moving ahead. The "witnessing" capacity of our mind is a hidden dimension of our intelligence beneath superficial thinking that is always present yet usually unrecognized, explains Christopher Baxter, founder of Inner Sky Yoga (personal communication). It is an inborn aspect of consciousness that has the ability to cognize both internal and external events in a way that is free of personal bias and self-interest. It is described as a nonjudgmental attention, independent of the usual burden of likes, dislikes, opinions, ignorance, worry, aggression, craving, fear, selfishness, and the boundless array of emotional obstacles. Yet this deep layer of attention is not unaffected, numb, indifferent, or unemotional coldness. It is warm-hearted unattachment that deeply cares and feels. Being unattached is being at peace with the polarities of life like loss and gain, fame and shame, and so forth.

Witness consciousness is cultivated and developed through meditation and practiced in daily living when one becomes an impartial observer of thoughts, feelings, emotions, and the events of living life—even while deeply sensitive to the suffering and happiness of ourselves and others. It is an unselfish awareness that removes us from the misperception that we are more important than others. As a result of letting go of addictive self-interest whereby we are indifferent to the needs of others, we relax and recognize the peace of seeing reality as it really is—that we have a place in the web of life, both giving and receiving.

Pure consciousness is beyond witness consciousness and exists when aspirations and efforts cease and our experience of ourselves expands beyond our small personal world, enabling us to recognize ourselves as unlimited awareness, infused with loving kindness and compassion.

Through actual experience, yoga nidra gives us solid practice developing witness consciousness and pure consciousness within the yoga nidra process. Results range from having the ability to manage stress on the practical level to feeling vibrantly alive, witnessing a profound indwelling sense of inner peace and clarity, even when we deeply feel the emotions—both happy and painful—of ourselves and others.

## Sam and Sallie's Stories

While at work, someone pushes Sam's buttons. Instantly, he flies off the handle. He shouts, "I'm so stressed! Can you believe what just happened?" Meanwhile, his heart is pumping and his blood pressure is rising as he chews out his coworker. The stress response has been automatically activated, and he is fighting mad. Instead, with study, practice, and the application of selected yoga principles like witness consciousness, he can learn how to catch himself by noticing his experience and reacting differently. He can notice, "Oh, here's stress and it's causing me to feel mad. Look at how I'm reacting. My shoulders are tense, my breathing is erratic, and I feel like yelling or hitting something." This newfound awareness causes a shift inside that opens up new options. He can consciously start putting a stop to the stress reaction and turn the relaxation response on by lengthening and deepening his exhalation. As his reactive desire to fight, expressed as anger, naturally dissipates, he can come back to the situation at hand from a new perspective that is fresh and free. He can then decide what action to take, if any, to resolve the problem.

In another case, Sallie can make better choices when she starts feeling stressed out from loneliness. Instead of identifying with the limiting belief "I'm so lonely," she can use the time-tested yogic principles included in this text to gradually gain access to her witness consciousness to impartially notice what is happening as it unfolds, step back from her habitual reactions, and clearly realize that "Here's loneliness and it's causing me stress. This is what it feels like. However, even though these thoughts and feelings are here, they're temporary and they do not reflect my true Self."

To get started using these new ways of responding to stress, practice the relaxation techniques taught in this book and in the audio recordings. This will help you know how to switch from feeling stressed to feeling in control. As these skills grow in strength, the time it takes between noticing feeling stressed and using your new tools for stress relief will shorten and become more effective.

## Release of False Identities

While stress management and relaxation are important, yoga sages believe that they are temporary fixes. Stress will always be experienced until we go through the process of discovering and releasing our misperceptions and false identities, and begin realizing our true Self.

Instead of falsely identifying with stress, like Sam's anger and Sallie's loneliness, each person can realize what they are experiencing with the understanding that it is temporary, and remember to call on their stress relief skills and inner resources. By accepting whatever happens, inner tension relaxes, stress automatically releases, and positive changes begin to happen naturally. This concept can be expressed like this:

Stressful Stimulus → Reaction

To

Stressful Stimulus → Awareness → Response

The teachings do not tell us to ignore or run away from anything. As a Catholic priest named Father Greg once said at a retreat, "The more you notice your thoughts and feelings, the more you witness, and the freer you become. The ordinary is the miracle. Altered mental states happen and begin to permeate your experience." Stress relieves itself. This can be accomplished through yoga nidra.

## It Takes Practice

The *Yoga Sutras* promise us that we will gain the profound understanding that our true essence goes far beyond our temporary physical, mental, and emotional components. Yoga Sutra I.14 says, "The practice of yoga will be firmly rooted when it is maintained consistently and with dedication over a long period" (Shearer 1982, 92). In *The Secret Power of Yoga*, Nischala Devi translates this verse as "*Abhyasa* (practice) is nurtured by a sustained, steady rhythm and a dedicated heart" (2007, 280).

You might be wondering how much practice is needed. Results often occur in stages. Right from the start, yoga nidra deactivates the stress reaction by activating the relaxation response. Feelings of peace and calmness are felt. Then you may notice that the more time you dwell in the yoga nidra state of conscious awareness (fully described later in this chapter), the more its qualities are available to you in day-to-day living. This is harmonizing for the body, mind, and spirit. It is like there is something that cushions you from stress so that the things that used to bother you are not so irritating. When stressful reactions do occur, we can intervene sooner, more positively, and productively. In addition, noticing goodness and beauty happens more often.

All these concepts and stress relief skills are practiced during yoga nidra. All three full yoga nidra exercises in this book—Relax, Reflect, and Revitalization—teach different methods to help you conquer physical stress and develop your capacity to quickly use your breath to calm down and clear your mind. In particular, the exercise found in chapter 4, based on progressive muscle relaxation, gives you the tools needed to wash stress away and directly experience the benefits of complete physical, mental, and emotional relaxation. Building on this, chapter 5 goes further into developing greater sensory awareness, observational skills, self-understanding, and intuitive wisdom; it uses the map of awareness based on the brain-body connection and the chakra system. Chapter 6 helps with gaining a handle on emotional stress and correcting false and limiting beliefs; it's based on the autogenic method of relaxation and the paradox of opposites. As you will find out in chapter 3, all of this is fortified with the unique power of using a resolve (*sankalpa*).

With ongoing practice, we begin to identify less with what is impermanent (thoughts, feelings, and actions, whether stressful or not) and pay more attention to what endures. This is not to say that we can ignore our daily responsibilities; instead, these responsibilities are understood and handled from a different perspective. Stress is relieved fundamentally and is transformed into awakened living.

## Many Yoga Paths Lead to Realizing the True Self

The ancient Yoga masters gave us many options and methods for accessing yoga's wisdom, teachings, and many benefits while accommodating and respecting our particular temperament, faith tradition, and learning style.

Each of the yogic paths named below is a valid and useful method of stress relief and Self-understanding. As a yoga slogan says, "The easy path is hard enough." So choose a path that is compatible with your temperament, needs, and interests.

**Karma yoga, a path of action:** serving others coupled with letting go of results; practicing selflessness; seeing the divine in others

**Jnana yoga, an intellectual path:** the study of philosophy and scriptures; Self-realization and understanding

**Bhakti yoga, the heart-centered path:** devotion through prayer, song, and worship

**Raja yoga, the mystical path of ethics/body/mind/spirit:** also referred to as *Ashtanga* yoga, described as an eight-faceted path leading to realizing our true Self in the Yoga Sutra II.29. These eight components, often referred to as limbs, are as follows:

## Social and Personal Ethics

1.  *Yamas:* the five tenets of living with respect for others, society, and the world are reverence for all life, non-harming (*ahimsa*), truthfulness (*satya*), integrity (*asteya*), moderation (*brahmacharya*), and nonattachment, lack of self-indulgence (*aparigraha*)

2.  *Niyamas:* the five tenets for personal living and attitudes toward oneself are cleanliness and purity (*shauca*), contentment (*samtosha*), self-discipline (*tapas*), Self-understanding (*svadhyaya*), and devotion to the Divine One—"Your will, not mine" (*Ishvara-pranidhana*)

## Hatha Yoga

3.  Asana: physical postures

4.  Pranayama: breathing techniques that enhance and direct prana, the vital life force

5.  Pratyahara: training and control of the senses

## Meditation

6. Dharana: steadiness of mind, concentration

7. Dhyana: meditation

8. Samadhi: contemplation, absorption, super-conscious state, union with Divine Consciousness

Yoga nidra falls under Raja (Ashtanga) yoga. Its associated teachings date back thousands of years and can be found in the wisdom teachings of the Upanishads, Classical Yoga, and in the Tantric tradition. In the 1970s, systematic, valid, and reliable ways of experiencing yoga nidra were identified. Since then, many others have developed additional methods, benefits, and applications for the yoga nidra experience.

Modern-day practitioners typically place their attention either outwardly on the physical postures and yoga breathing or inwardly on meditation. What is often ignored is the pratyahara stage in between that connects what is external with what is internal. This cuts short the benefits of the postures and makes meditation more challenging. Practiced during yoga nidra, pratyahara plays a vital role in making this transition.

## Controlling the Senses (Pratyahara)

In Raja yoga, the control and the withdrawal of the senses are referred to as pratyahara. Yoga nidra is a technique used to redirect sensory awareness from an external focus to an internal one. Pratyahara is not withdrawal from living life. Instead of being an escape, the process of pratyahara expands our awareness and we become more sensitized to living life more authentically. With practice, we learn to notice our external circumstances as well as our internal thoughts, perceptions, and emotional reactions while they are happening in a nonjudgmental and nonevaluative manner. As awareness increases, we move from being reactionary to stressors and sensory experiences (what we see, hear, feel, taste, perceive) to becoming increasingly more responsive. Instead of being driven by stress, past conditioning, and opinions, we have a longer fuse and the opportunity to respond more appropriately.

Our senses and sensory awareness surely have their place in daily life, but they distract us from our true Self. Senses are temporary phenomenon, whereas our true Self is permanent.

Sri Swami Satchidananda further clarifies this in his translation and commentary on *The Yoga Sutras of Patanjali* (1978). In his book, he explains that the senses are a gateway that allows external influences to come into the mind. They serve like a mirror. When the senses are turned outward, they reflect what is outside and transfer sensory experiences to the mind, causing mental restlessness.

## Mary's Story

Mary struggles with sensory distractions on a regular basis. She is easily distracted whether she is busy doing something or sitting for meditation. For example, she notices a tempting smell. Her mouth begins to water. If she is not careful, she will react by eating, whether or not she is hungry. With greater sensory awareness, she can notice the smell and continue with whatever she is doing. Another option is to notice the tempting smell, determine whether she is hungry, and decide whether to eat something.

During pratyahara, our senses are no longer outwardly active (noticing sounds, smells, etc.). When this happens, our attention naturally turns inward. When turned inward, the mirror reflects the inner light, the pure light of inner peace (Satchidananda 1978).

When awareness of our external senses withdraws, we are easily led into a natural state of inner concentration, contemplation, and absorption. This is meditation. The experiential exercises in future chapters will skillfully guide us toward this. In time and with practice, this type of perception, insight, and sensitivity becomes the norm rather than the exception. A felt sense of inner peace becomes pervasive, even under stress. In other words, having a felt sense of peacefulness goes beyond hoping, relying on the imagination, or thinking to having a direct bodily experience and an inner awareness of peace. It is like having an inner knowing and "feeling it in your bones."

Some forms of meditation rely on concentration techniques and are quite effective. However, concentration gets in the way of yoga nidra. In mindfulness meditation techniques, the focus is to stay awake and notice, observe, and remain undisturbed when thoughts, words, feelings, beliefs, sensory experiences, and images appear and disappear. Mindfulness is a beneficial stage of yoga nidra that is experienced and surpassed.

## Yoga Nidra Is "Yogic Sleep"

Most people who suffer from stress do not sleep well and feel exhausted. In fact, stress is one of the leading causes of insomnia, and a vicious cycle can get cranked up. Not only is it frustrating, sleep deprivation increases cortisol, the stress hormone, and cortisol can lead to insomnia. Lack of sleep may lead to weight gain, substance abuse, irritability, lowered performance, and a higher risk for accidents due to slower reaction time. It can contribute to depression and anxiety (Talbot 2011). In other words, more stress.

The methods used for experiencing yoga nidra can be used to help you fall asleep. Taking time to relax your body, mind, and emotions will first enable you to sleep soundly, since daily stresses are not carried with you into sleep. Yoga nidra used as a sleep aid, however, should not be confused with the actual experience of yoga nidra itself. Be careful or it will become hard to experience full yoga nidra, as you'll make it a habit of falling asleep instead.

In yoga nidra, we ultimately experience what is called "yogic sleep," which is not like typical sleep. The delta brain wave state we eventually experience during advanced yoga nidra is like being in deep sleep with one big difference: our awareness remains alert and awake rather than unconscious. In one of its earlier phases, it feels similar to how you feel when you are either just falling asleep or are on the verge of waking up. Most of us are not accustomed to noticing this transitional experience between being awake and asleep or realize its value and importance. Not paying attention to this potent place of consciousness is like not noticing the pauses between each inhalation and exhalation. These pauses are vital to respiration, but they are rarely noticed or valued. Without these pauses, breathing would stop.

Learning to stay on the verge of being awake and asleep is a very important, powerful, and fertile doorway, or midpoint. This still point is called the *madhya*, or center. Sally Kempton describes it as a state of awareness in which we enter "the inner space where we experience our connection to the whole." She also says this "fractional pause in the flow of the breath or in the flow of thoughts then opens out into the vastness of Consciousness." It is "the space of the heart" (Durgananda 2002, 34).

Even though yoga nidra is not a substitute for sleep, it is believed that one hour of practice is equivalent to four hours of regular sleep (Goel 2001). This is because we consciously go through all the brain wave stages experienced during sleep but in a compressed time frame.

## Understanding Atma and the Koshas

The practice of yoga nidra is based on understanding and experiencing the relationship between the koshas and the Atma and putting this knowledge to use.

Since ancient times, Yoga masters have taught that we are multidimensional beings by nature. Early on, they realized that we are composed of five different dimensions (the koshas) that are metaphorically referred to as "bodies." They include our physical body that is composed of flesh and bones; our energetic body that is composed of our life force; our mental body composed of our thoughts, emotions, feelings, and beliefs; our intuitive wisdom body; and our blissful body. The koshas were first described about 3,000 years ago in a text known as the *Taittiriya Upanishad*. We will refer to the koshas as layers, even though they can also be referred to as sheaths, coverings, envelopes, or facets. Our essential Self is expressed outwardly through the koshas.

# Atma: Our True, Transcendental, and Essential Self

The Atma denotes the source of our transcendental, true Self. When accessed, there is a spontaneous and genuine inner knowing and remembrance of the universal Presence that can be characterized as Oneness, Spirit, God, Goddess, Buddha-nature, or other portrayals that realize the Atman. Yoga masters believe the Atma is eternal, pure, boundless, and unchanging.

You might be wondering why it is so easy to feel stressed and so difficult to get in touch with this inner source of unending peace, unconditional joy, and wisdom. Here are a few reasons to consider:

- Our essential Self is overshadowed by the koshas. It is covered up by our bodily needs and a variety of sensual, emotional, and mental attractions and distractions. Yoga nidra peels away these layers, enabling us to experience our essential Self even when in the midst of chaos, ill health, or stress.

- We mistakenly seek out temporary pleasure rather than enduring happiness and joy.

- We expect joy to feel like winning a gold medal at the Olympics rather than experiencing it as a subtle sense of inner joy, peacefulness, contentment, and compassion.

- Many of us have been wounded and scarred, thus coloring our thoughts, feelings, and reactions in stressful ways.

- False and unrealistic expectations cloud our thinking.

- Rather than living in the present moment nonjudgmentally, the past and future dominate our attention.

- Our past actions, good and bad, influence our current perceptions and actions and can sidetrack us from knowing our inner truth. Yoga philosophy calls this *karma*; it is the principle of cause and effect or "What you sow is what you reap."

■ In *Pocketful of Miracles*, Joan Borysenko writes, "In spite of our inner drive to wake up to our essential nature, there is another force of mind working to keep us asleep—the ego. As a psychologist, I think of this aspect of personality as the 'conditioned self.' It arises in response to the conditions of life that threaten to separate us from love. As we grow up, we don a variety of masks that we show to the world in an attempt to be lovable, or at least powerful. The masks help us feel safe. Paradoxically, they are informed by fear and keep us separate from the only true source of love—the Divine Mind. In spiritual systems, the fear-based conditioned self is called the ego. This is different from ego as it is used in psychological parlance to denote a healthy, independent sense of self" (1994, 35).

Yoga nidra gives us techniques, via the koshas, to understand and go through the above list to reveal and experience our true Self and feel free.

## The Koshas

Since Yoga masters believe that the following five layers hide our essential Self, it is important to understand them. We incorrectly believe the illusion that these five layers make up who we are. This illusion is referred to as *maya*. But it is the Atma that makes up who we truly are. Even though the koshas are described independently and distinctly, in reality the lines distinguishing them are subtle and interdependent, like in a rainbow. Additionally, there are straightforward as well as sophisticated relationships among them. The koshas work together interactively and influence each other negatively, neutrally, or positively.

The stress reaction is experienced holistically, not just physically, emotionally, or mentally. In other words, the koshas come into play when our buttons get pushed. For instance, our shoulders might get tight, our breath becomes shallow, we start feeling anxious, and our thoughts might run wild. This could lead to a sleepless night or worse. Therefore, to take care of stress, a multidimensional approach is needed.

One role of yoga nidra is to help us identify our issues and to relax, heal, and transcend the koshas to experience our true Self. Through a systematic process, we can overcome the illusion—maya—that our body, mind, emotions, and even our intuitive and joyful nature are what are real by putting them to rest temporarily. As this happens, the process of withdrawing the senses (pratyahara) naturally happens as attention moves inward and past each of these layers. The yoga nidra process brings us profound relaxation and renewal, allowing us to be inwardly reflective. It is meditative, revitalizing, and enables us to remember our true Self.

## Anna Maya Kosha

The anna maya kosha refers to our physical makeup, including all our muscles, joints, flesh, bones, blood, and vital organs. It is the tangible material that makes up our body. It can be seen, touched, and felt. It is our anatomy and physiology. The term "anna" refers to the "food body."

The relaxation response is experienced in yoga nidra by systematically and progressively relaxing every muscle in the material body. This first stage of relaxation results in a very heavy physical sensation in the body. It feels extremely calming and delightful. Useful relaxation skills are developed that can be applied whenever needed during stressful times.

## Prana Maya Kosha

The prana maya kosha refers to the universal life force that infuses all creation. The Chinese system refers to this life force as *chi* and the Japanese call it *ki*. This life force is what activates our physical body, energizes us with vital energy, and fuels our subtle anatomy. Our subtle anatomy is composed of our energy centers, called *chakras*, and energy channels called *nadis* (pronounced *NAH-deez*). Together they work through meditation, affirmations, and the breath to rebalance the energy system during yoga nidra.

57

Under stress, respiration changes and the breath becomes shallow, rapid, and irregular instead of smooth, deep, and regular. Likewise, even under calm conditions, just changing your breathing pattern by making the inhalation longer than the exhalation can produce the stress response.

Special breathing techniques are used for relaxing, settling, and reviving oneself energetically, since prana is primarily cultivated and directed by the breath. The relaxation response is reinforced. Practicing the breathing techniques can correct poor breathing habits. These techniques can be practiced anytime for instant stress relief. The healthful benefits of breathing properly will begin to spill over into daily living and can keep the stress reaction at bay, especially when full respiration becomes natural and automatic again. A variety of helpful breathing techniques are described in appendices 2 and 3.

When the prana maya kosha relaxes during yoga nidra, a feeling of inner stillness accompanies the muscular heaviness already being experienced. Breathing naturally deepens, slows down, and becomes subtler.

## Mano Maya Kosha

"*Manas*" means "mind" in Sanskrit. This layer is composed of the thoughts, concepts, beliefs, emotions, and feelings that make up our personality. This aspect of ourselves can either support our well-being or trigger stress.

Under stress, thoughts go astray and set off an emotional reaction. Insecurities, fear, anger, and confusion can result. The reverse is also true. Faulty thoughts and irrational feelings cause stress as well.

During this third stage of relaxation and renewal, mental and emotional stress is steadily lifted through a variety of techniques, such as guided imagery and visualization. As this happens, the sensation of physical heaviness naturally lifts, and a buoyant feeling that is light and freeing occurs. It often feels like you are floating on air.

When you train rather than control your thoughts, faulty and limiting beliefs, inappropriate emotional reactions, and unhelpful thoughts are less likely to occur throughout the day. The more the mano maya kosha stage is practiced during yoga nidra, the more mindfulness takes root and becomes available more regularly.

### Vijnana Maya Kosha

"Vijnana" can be defined as our intuitive sense, and direct awareness that spontaneously arises. The vijnana maya kosha frees us from limiting beliefs, elicits mental clarity, heightens intuition, and increases creativity. The vijnana maya kosha gives us the vantage point of being an impartial witness and provides us with a depth of wisdom and understanding that is transcendental. As this stage of yoga nidra is practiced with regularity, these qualities start showing up at other times. Actions and decisions become more positive, productive, and wise, lowering stress levels.

Under stress, we tend to become reactive rather than responsive. We stay identified with our limiting thoughts and beliefs. Intuitive wisdom and insights are lost or ignored.

When the thinking mind comes to rest, intuitive wisdom reveals itself and awareness expands. This is the fourth stage of relaxation. By this time, your body has completely relaxed physically and energetically. In addition, a sense of total mental and emotional relaxation occurs. A temporary sense of detachment and freedom from all your worldly cares and concerns arises. Since nothing is holding you down, a sense of timelessness and weightlessness is experienced.

### Ananda Maya Kosha

"Ananda" is translated as "joy" or "bliss." This is our most subtle layer. It consists of our innate qualities including inner peace, joy, wholeness, and contentment. These enduring qualities are intrinsic to our true Self and independent of possessions or conditions of any type.

When we lose this realization, it is a double-edged sword. Not only does it cause stress, we cannot experience these underlying qualities in their purest form.

Profound relaxation and an awareness of being that goes far beyond the mindbody happen during this stage. In this final stage of relaxation, absolute stillness is present and a state of joyful well-being is pervasive. Timelessness and spaciousness is experienced. With ongoing practice, inner peace and joy eventually begin to permeate living. When having to handle stress, a deep reservoir of inner knowing is present; there's the understanding that stress is temporary and does not reflect the bigger picture of who you really are and what is truly important. All these steps and stages help you remember your inner core and true Self.

The ananda maya kosha opens into experiencing the Atma. This stage is indescribable, but let me try. It is experiencing the art of stepping back with a deeper perspective, even beyond the witness consciousness. This gives us the sense of resting in oneself with a profound sense of contentment and fulfillment. There is absolutely no sense of suffering or discontent. Furthermore, there is a heartfelt connection with everyone and everything. Total satisfaction is felt that goes beyond the pleasures that come and go.

## The Labyrinth of the Koshas and Atma

The layers of the koshas are traditionally shown as either Russian dolls nesting within each other or depicted graphically as a series of concentric circles surrounding a center point (Atma). The center is surrounded by the innermost ring, which represents the bliss body (ananda maya kosha). The outermost ring represents the physical layer (anna maya kosha), with the other layers positioned in between. The idea of concentric circles implies a definite division and separation between the layers and does not allow a way to naturally journey from one layer to the next. Furthermore, from my experience as a teacher and practitioner, it has become clear that the boundaries between the koshas are really more fuzzy and porous—they interact with one another. Therefore, using an image of a labyrinth and its journey is a better metaphor to represent the koshas and the Atma, in my opinion (see illustration).

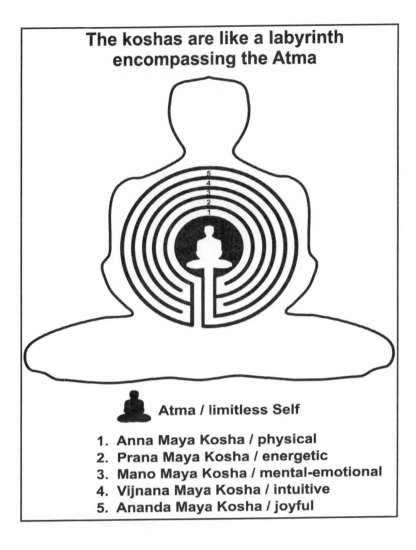

**The koshas are like a labyrinth encompassing the Atma**

- Atma / limitless Self
1. **Anna Maya Kosha / physical**
2. **Prana Maya Kosha / energetic**
3. **Mano Maya Kosha / mental-emotional**
4. **Vijnana Maya Kosha / intuitive**
5. **Ananda Maya Kosha / joyful**

A labyrinth is a single, one-way path into a center and then back out. It is not a confusing maze with twists and turns to figure out. Labyrinths can be viewed or walked meditatively as a tool for personal, psychological, and spiritual transformation. Serving as a living metaphor, the labyrinth experience is known for helping to remember one's true Self by connecting us to the depths of our soul. Taken one step at a time, it depicts the journey of following a well-traveled and proven path with the understanding that every experience is unique. All you have to do is start at the opening of the entrance and follow the path. Use your finger to trace the path from the entrance at the bottom into the center and back out again in the illustration to familiarize yourself with this path.

Think of the labyrinth's journey as having the following parts for a complete experience. To start, an intention is set with an open mind and heart. The walk inward to the center is dedicated to shedding whatever is unnecessary. While inside, the center's mysterious and intuitive qualities can create the opportunity to receive whatever insights are ready to be revealed. Returning after being in the center (centered) is the next step. This is a time for further reflection and for taking the revitalizing gifts discovered along the way back into your life. The possibilities are endless and might include healing, self-understanding, and clarity. Upon returning, feelings of renewal and revitalization are often felt.

Balancing the koshas and putting them to rest through yoga nidra is much like walking a labyrinth. A similar three-part journey is taken to overcome stress and to experience your essential, peaceful, soulful Self. This happens by going through the steps of releasing stress through the koshas, dwelling in the center, and then returning. A sankalpa is used at the start and finish, as can be done in setting an intention prior to walking a labyrinth. Developing and using a sankalpa is detailed in chapter 3.

As is true with both a labyrinth and yoga nidra, you have to take the journey, navigate the distractions, and correct false beliefs; then you can enjoy basking in the center. Finally, in making the deliberate transition back from the center to normal wakefulness, it is important to bring all the benefits of your experience back with you for yourself and for the sake of others.

Using the labyrinth to symbolize the koshas and the Atma implies an orderly, systematic, multifaceted path. Practicing yoga nidra magnifies the likelihood of experiencing a stress-free zone of oneness and feeling truly centered. It is entirely possible to discover for yourself the contrast between the changeability of your physical, mental, and emotional nature and the enduring, never-changing quality of your true essence on this journey. Once this happens, you will be capable of handling stress with greater ease and have the understanding that stress, no matter its source, is temporary and does not reflect your true identity. Rather than being caught up in the drama, you are able to wholeheartedly respond to life more mindfully and with greater ease and intellect. Additionally, you will have the opportunity to receive guidance from your wisdom source (vijnana), have the cognitive capacity and understanding to move ahead with your mind and emotions in balance (mano) with the energy needed (prana) to embody (anna) right action. The more steady and comfortable you become in the practice of yoga nidra, the more readily these skills will be available for you. These abilities also become easier and swifter as well.

## What to Remember

- Millions of practicing yogis and the general public are finally realizing that yoga is much more than physical postures. It holds the secret for improving your health and gaining relaxed energy by relieving stress and experiencing your true Self (Atma), which is described as peaceful, loving, indelible, joyful, and luminous. Layers, called koshas, cover this elegance. The role of Yoga is to shed stress and reveal these qualities. No matter what is going on around us or within us, the central qualities of our true Self are always present. Our thoughts and feelings often disturb the peace that is constantly there. When the thinking mind becomes still with pure awareness, peace is automatically revealed, even in the midst of chaos, ill health, or stress. This suggests that a living duality exists. It is a kind of perfect imperfection. There is the objective reality of daily living, and another underlying reality that embraces the universal truths that are present in the great wisdom traditions, including Yoga. These levels of reality occupy the same space. Perhaps, then, it is not so much a matter of either/or but of both/and.

- Yoga nidra is a valuable tool for your stress relief toolbox. It is both relaxing and healing, and it contains a pathway to Self-understanding. Yoga nidra is a state of consciousness and not a particular posture or technique. Relaxation exercises, breathing techniques, meditations, guided imagery techniques, and visualizations are simply the tools used to experience yoga nidra. A single method for reaching yoga nidra does not exist. No one owns it. It is universal.

- Yoga nidra is extremely relaxing, energizing, and empowering; it decreases physical tension and activates the relaxation response; it replaces internal commotion and limiting beliefs with inner peace, clear thinking, and enhanced, intuitive awareness; it feels blissfully like heaven on Earth; it's a pathway to the Self; and it only works if practiced—knowing about it is not enough.

- Living life is more than handling stress. It is about living a joyful life (ananda) with meaning and purpose (dharma) and reaching Self-realization (atma-jnana). Yoga nidra gives us a straightforward pathway and method for doing so—and it feels truly joyful.

- Lean toward steadiness and ease.

## Chapter 3

# Getting Started: How to Practice Yoga Nidra

This chapter gives important instructions for practicing yoga nidra. Subsequent chapters provide specific practices for experiencing it.

Yoga nidra gives us the direct experience of stress relief and the relaxation response. It provides us with a practical process for creating the conditions needed to experience and benefit from our thoughts and feelings—but from a different point of reference. Using a resolve, called a *sankalpa*, brings another dimension of benefits to life—your life!

As a quick review, yoga nidra shows us the importance of being non-attached. Instead of identifying with our circumstances, thoughts, and feelings, it teaches us to identify with what is unchanging. Stress can be viewed as impermanent and temporary, even if it does not feel that way in the moment. Yoga nidra helps us learn to become objective and aware of what is going on in and around us, and to respond to it all mindfully rather than reacting out of our habits and conditioning. This type of awareness, often referred to as *witness consciousness*, allows for the presence and flow of thoughts and feelings; but instead of identifying with them, we identify with our real Self. Yoga masters believe that stress management and relaxation training are temporary fixes. We will always experience stress until we can eventually identify with our true Self, or *Atma*. This is a gradual process and takes time and patience. With dedicated practice, peace and happiness can become our baseline.

The more our skills and abilities develop through practice, the more likely we will respond mindfully—aware of our thoughts, sensing our feelings and emotions, and receptive to our intuitive wisdom. This perspective enables us to take appropriate action, solve problems, and reduce stress. As practice deepens, we can experience the Atma, the place within that is always stress-free and unchanging.

Furthermore, yoga nidra gives us the healing and direct experience of feeling calm and joyful. This takes place not only during our formal practice of yoga nidra but in daily living as well. We learn how to remain at peace even in the swirl of our thoughts or in the midst of an emotional reaction.

There is only one hitch: We have got to do it! There is no better teacher than experience. Reading and knowing about yoga nidra will not cut it. It has to be experienced. The taste of an orange can be described forever, but until you eat one you will never truly know its flavor, texture, aroma, and juiciness. The same goes for feeling the benefits of yoga nidra.

Like anything worthwhile, devoting ample time and effort to your practice is important. The beauty is that practicing counteracts tension, giving the feeling of being calm during practice. It frees up energy by neutralizing limiting thoughts, beliefs, and feelings. All this starts to carry over into daily living so that we feel more at ease and energized in general. As one yoga slogan goes, "Take it easy—not lazy."

## Understanding and Setting a Sankalpa

Another important distinguishing aspect of yoga nidra that sets it apart from other stress relief and relaxation training methods is the use of a sankalpa. This Sanskrit word is often translated as "a resolve" or "resolution." Some think of it as an intention. Rod Stryker, founder of Para Yoga, explains that "*kalpa* means 'vow,' or 'the rule to be followed above all other rules... *San* refers to a connection with the highest truth. Sankalpa, then, is a vow and commitment we make to support our highest truth" (McGonigal 2010–2011). We use the word "sankalpa" in this book because using an English equivalent like setting a resolve or intention does not fully capture the meaning and intent of this concept.

Sankalpa also refers to an important part of the process in a yoga nidra session.

## A Sankalpa Helps Make Positive Changes

How many times have you sincerely promised yourself that you were going to make some positive change, to no avail? Perhaps it was to make lifestyle improvements such as lowering your stress levels by improving your nutrition and exercise habits. Maybe it was to develop helpful characteristics like being more calm, patient, courageous, or less judgmental. Another might have been to establish and follow through on having a positive and meaningful life direction. Making changes such as these is tough.

Our day-to-day frame of consciousness (beta brain waves) makes it extremely difficult to make and maintain these good intentions because they crash into our long-term conditioning, habits, and social pressures. Through no fault of your own, your mind is simply not very receptive to making these changes. During yoga nidra, we knowingly, consciously, and consecutively experience a range of different types of brain wave levels: alpha, theta, and delta frequencies. The level reached at the end of practice is *very* receptive to change. When we implant a sankalpa in the subconscious mind, useless thoughts and behaviors *can* be weeded out, and the conditions are created for significant and transformative change to take root and grow.

Yogis must have understood and applied the concept of *neuroplasticity* long ago. "Neuro" refers to the nerve cells of the brain, and "plasticity" refers to the brain's ability to reorganize and restructure itself after training or practice. The brain never stops changing as the nerve cells (neurons) and other structures in it adjust and respond to new situations and changes in the environment. New neural connections are made that are related to making changes in behavior, thinking, and emotions *throughout* the entire lifespan, not just during infancy (Doidge 2007). This helps explain why using a sankalpa during yoga nidra is so effective for making lasting changes *if* the same one is used and practiced regularly.

By the way, there are built-in contradictions to appreciate. Yoga philosophers believe that your essential Self is already whole, joyful, and peaceful. At the same time there is another aspect of yourself that is in the process of growing and developing, encouraging you to become the person you want to be and to do what is important with your life.

The choice is entirely yours with respect to the type and quality of sankalpa made. Instead of someone else—a friend, teacher, or therapist—telling you what to choose, it is totally up to you. You are given the opportunity to let a sankalpa arise from deep inside yourself during yoga nidra.

## Lynn's Story

I started practicing yoga after I had quit drinking for two years. I began using a sankalpa six months ago. I chose "I am content." Six weeks ago, I added "I am confident."

Behind all this is that I seem to doubt myself with decisions at work, in my marriage, and in relationships with family. It's stressful. I am tired of second-guessing myself and wondering if I should have said or done something else. I also felt dissatisfied with many aspects of my life. I want to be happy, patient, and fulfilled.

In using my sankalpa, I hoped to find inner strength, confidence, and joy. I use it during my yoga nidra practice at home and in class. I also repeat it if my mind wanders during class, when I take walks or garden, and when slipping into self-doubt. It helped me get past the usual barriers and resistance the mind usually puts up for protection and to resist change. Yoga nidra allowed my resolve to stick.

I did gain more confidence at work and have been better at not doubting my abilities, progress, or decisions. At home, I've made some decisions about where I want to be in my marriage and my perspective on it, and I've communicated what I expect to him. Before, I was just floating along with the status quo and silently trying to deal with it on my own.

I still have moments of impatience, but I'm finding happiness in small things like a beautiful sunset, my garden, my cats, my friends, my time, and the smile on my daughter's face. I am happier, period. Are there spots for improvement? Of course, but I am committed to working on them when I can and am ready. I am not beating myself up about it anymore.

## Types of Sankalpas

Choose something personally meaningful, even noble. Sure, you can have one to bring about short-term results ("Get me through this stressful day") but having a sankalpa that really feels right and solidifies your deepest desires will generate both short- and long-term results. Take your time. Why rush into this? Some ideas for consideration are:

- A positive virtue or characteristic: calmness, kindness, patience, acceptance, courage, confidence, and so on

- A change in behavior

- A specific intention that can guide you during the next year or so

- Something meaningful to do with your life: establishment and support for your life direction

Rather than becoming overwhelmed by all the possible qualities and potential changes you would like to make, choose only one to focus on. Having a sankalpa is just like picking up a string of beautiful gems. When you pick up the first gem, the others naturally follow. Let's use kindness as an example. Kindness is a virtue that goes a long way toward making positive changes and getting stress relief. Kindness serves as the primary jewel. Practicing kindness in general would naturally lead to being kinder to oneself by making better lifestyle choices for stress relief such as improving nutrition and exercise habits. Being kinder would facilitate the cultivation of patience and understanding.

Furthermore, acceptance of oneself and others, gratitude, and peace of mind would naturally follow. Meanwhile, making all these changes would be simplified and less stressful because the focus is simply centered on kindness. In other words, kindness facilitates stress relief and a whole lot more.

## Susan's Story

Susan's job was no longer satisfying. The low pay and long hours were stressful, and her boss wanted her to start doing things that went against her values. She was hesitant to make any job changes since she had a kid in college, another in high school, and one in middle school. All this pressure caused her a lot of frustration and confusion. In addition, Susan's doctor was on her back about improving her diet and getting more exercise to help her diabetes and hypertension. She often felt torn between her family, work, and personal responsibilities. Her worries added to her irritability. It was getting harder and harder for her to get to sleep and stay asleep.

Susan decided to set a sankalpa. She wisely realized that simultaneously tackling a job search, making nutritional and exercise improvements, and striving for life balance, happiness, and mental clarity would be overwhelming, confusing, and stressful. She knew that setting a sankalpa wasn't supposed to be an additional stressor.

What pressed Susan the most was getting a new job. Yet, instead of setting a sankalpa such as "I want a new job," she chose "abundance." That way, abundance could come as a new job or in another form. Who knew? Maybe a windfall would come her way. Perhaps changes to her current job would give her the satisfaction she was seeking. She lacked the extra time and energy needed for all this to happen. She was skeptical, to say the least.

Susan decided to resign from her job and start a job search in earnest. She said her sankalpa, "I have abundance," each time she practiced yoga nidra. During her job interviews Susan also held the *kubera mudra* (see appendix 1) for achieving goals. Within a few months, she had three job offers to choose from. She is amazed that more job offers are still coming her way.

Improving her diet and getting more exercise were also changes that Susan needed to make for her health and overall energy. She wondered how she was going to find the time, energy, and willpower to make these changes, especially with a new job and all her other responsibilities. She realized she could stay with abundance as her sankalpa, and benefit from abundant time and resources for the lifestyle improvements needed for abundant health. However, she chose "balance" as her sankalpa for the next phase of her life. She sought to find balance in diet and exercise, as well as in her home and work life. She found that the lifestyle improvements she was making also lowered her stress levels. And she was sleeping better too.

## Steps to Set Your Sankalpa

First, go back to the Assess Your Stress questionnaire in chapter 1 and to any notes you made in your journal. Review what you had checked and written down.

Next, reflect on the *opposite* qualities that would be a remedy to the symptoms of stress you checked off. For example, if you marked fear as a symptom, being brave or courageous are potential opposites as remedies to consider.

Look for trends next. Do one or two qualities stand out? Is there a common thread that ties most everything together? Could there be something that simply seems right? Keep in mind that making intellectual resolves rarely yields results, so find a balance between thinking it through and letting it come to you intuitively. Feel it out. Know that there is also time set aside during the yoga nidra process itself to allow a sankalpa to reveal itself rather than trying to figure it out intellectually.

Word your sankalpa briefly, sincerely, positively, and in the present tense. Say it as if it were already true. Back it up with gratitude along with your inner will.

Sample sankalpas include:

> "I am kind" or "My true nature is kindness" or "I am grateful for my kindness."

> "I am calm and peaceful."

> "I embrace all of who I am. I enjoy life fully."

> "I am trusting" or "My true nature is trusting."

> "I see the big picture of my life and move forward joyfully."

> "I am contentment personified."

> "I am healthy and well."

> "My true nature is joyful."

If using the phrase "I am" seems too far-fetched or demanding, try adding "more and more" at the beginning so the statement doesn't feel like such a stretch; it also makes room for incremental changes. For example, "More and more, I am courageous."

Write down your sankalpa in your journal. Then list some other qualities that will likely stem from your sankalpa.

Reinforce your sankalpa with the kubera yoga mudra (see appendix 1). (Mudras are yoga postures done with specific hand gestures rather than with the whole body.) The kubera mudra can be used during yoga nidra when saying your sankalpa as well as at other times such as while walking, praying, and meditating.

## Using Sankalpas During Yoga Nidra

Sankalpas are said silently at the beginning and end of each yoga nidra practice. Put your heart into it. Use your senses to imagine what it would actually feel like if it were already true.

It is important to be consistent. Changing it too often or having too many sankalpas frequently breeds confusion and diminishes effectiveness. Even though you may see results early on, give it a chance to fully manifest and make a difference in your life in multiple ways. Trust in it.

Remembering your sankalpa right when you are waking up or going to sleep is a potent time to reinforce the qualities being developed. The types of brain wave activities taking place during those times are especially receptive for this.

## Carol's Story

When given the opportunity to come up with a sankalpa several months ago, "courage" was the first thing that came to my mind.

I've always sketched, drawn, and painted. My work always felt too personal/not good enough/blah blah blah to ever share with anyone else. However, I have slowly—courageously—been showing my paintings to artists in a private online group. I found myself gradually starting to share them with friends and family and even on my own Facebook page. Then one day a local artist asked me if I wanted my own art show. It turns out she's the new art curator at a gallery downtown. Holy cow!

It was pretty exciting for a few days thinking about the possibility of an art show—until I got word that it had fallen through. At first I thought, "Screw sankalpas! My work is crap, I'm never going to paint again..." That brief, sad pity party was interrupted when this BIG BOOMING VOICE came through loud and clear: "What is *wrong* with you?! Show some of that COURAGE." I was back in the studio that afternoon.

A few weeks later, I got up my courage again to take a few days off from my "real job" to attend an out-of-town workshop offered by a well-known artist. I was really freaking out because she is known for doing strange things during workshops—like drumming and walking on coals—and I am very shy. So I stepped into my "courage" and practiced lots of yogic breathing to get up my nerve to go.

The first day left me so overwhelmed I just wanted to go home. Instead, I used my breath, kept centered and present, and showed up for day two. That's when the amazing magic started. After the workshop, the teacher shared her thoughts with us. What she said about me was, "I was honored to be in the presence of an artist who is so beyond amazing that, in my opinion, all she needs to do is paint and paint some more. At some point someone from New York will find her and she will be famous." Never in a gazillion years would I have predicted what she said about me.

Those sankalpas should come with a warning: "Caution: Sankalpas Can Be Life Changing!"

## Establishing a Regular Yoga Nidra Practice

Yoga Sutra I.14 reads: "The practice of yoga will be firmly [grounded] when it is maintained consistently and with dedication over a long time" (Shearer 1982, 92). And the Bhagavad Gita 2.40 says: "No effort is wasted and no gain is ever lost when on this path; even a little practice will shelter you from sorrow and protect you from the greatest fear" (Lusk 2005b, 175). Here are more tried-and-true tips for getting your yoga nidra practice started—and keeping it going. Being prepared and knowing what to expect will accelerate your progress.

**There are many right ways to practice.** The basic principles for your practice are to listen, participate, stay awake and aware, and welcome whatever happens. Otherwise, there are no wrong ways of practicing. As you will soon learn, there are many options available for entering yoga nidra, including the method used, the physical position chosen for practice, and the time of day and length of practice time. You are in charge.

**Choose the time of day wisely. Yoga nidra is a complete practice and can be done anytime.** If you practice during the day, you will feel a deep state of restfulness while doing it, and you will feel energized when you are finished. The result is nothing like the groggy feeling after taking an afternoon nap. Instead, it serves as a refreshing pick-me-up. You will find that if you practice at bedtime, it will help you fall asleep; just remember that you are using the method to fall asleep rather than to experience yoga nidra itself. If you practice hatha yoga either on your own or at a class, yoga nidra is practiced after the postures. Likewise, it is a wonderful prelude to meditation.

**A regular practice is much better than a sporadic one.** Maximum benefits occur when yoga nidra is done regularly. Ideally, it should be practiced daily, especially if you are under a load of stress or are sick; it facilitates progress remarkably. But several times a week is also very beneficial. Regular practice will benefit you in the short run as well as in the long term. The more often yoga nidra is experienced, the more its qualities will be available to you in daily living. Overcoming stress with relaxation will become much easier. You will remember to adjust your breathing to a healthy pace more often, and you will begin noticing that relaxed breathing is happening more and more on its own. Stress-producing thoughts, feelings, and actions will diminish. As mental clarity, emotional stability, and enhanced intuition improve, problem solving and creativity will increase. Feelings of acceptance, appreciation, and peace will become the norm.

**Vary the amount of practice as needed.** A complete yoga nidra session averages thirty minutes but can range from fifteen minutes to up to an hour. Whatever amount of time you dedicate to it is well worth it. Let your own experience guide you. Feeling refreshed and renewed after practicing yoga nidra is one of its goals. In other words, you may need to either shorten or lengthen your pracice to receive the desired effect.

**There is no need to hurry.** Give yourself all the time needed to thoroughly get to know each of the stages. For example, spend your time relaxing physically until you are comfortable with that stage. The next time, dedicate your time to relaxing energetically, and so on. This principle can also be applied when you are being guided in a group session or by a recording. In other words, you can stay with your own experience for as long as you feel engaged with it, and tune back in when you are ready. As one yoga slogan goes, "Start off slowly—and taper off."

**When time is short, pace yourself.** In reality, it can be difficult to take time out for yourself when stress is high and time is short—a combination that makes it too easy to forfeit regular practice. However, stressful times are when practicing is most important. Start with the amount of time you have available. If you need to shorten your practice, it is better to omit sections than to rush through your experience. Get to know and experience each of the stages one at a time instead of trying to fit them all in during one session. In addition, there are some quick and easy relaxation, breathing, and meditation options in appendices 2 and 3.

**Repeating the same yoga nidra sequence is very beneficial.** You will experience continuing layers of depth as your needs, experience, and capacity changes.

**Let your expectations go.** At times, you will have an amazing experience and will want to repeat it. Unfortunately, trying to make something happen again will not work. Learn to trust and accept whatever *does* happen. You are still benefiting even if you fall asleep or it sometimes seems like nothing is happening.

**Choose a practice method that suits your needs.** Consider trying all of these options until you find the one that resonates with you:

- *Practice with a teacher.* If practicing under the guidance of a teacher, choose someone with experience. Inquire about his or her background and training. Whether in a group or one on one, a qualified teacher can customize your experience depending on your needs and skill level. Pacing can be adjusted, and pertinent reminders can be added for maximum effectiveness. You will be less likely to fall asleep and more likely to experience yoga nidra. It will also afford you the opportunity to discuss and process your experience. Practicing with other people is motivating and will help you establish a consistent practice.

- *Practice with an audio recording.* Recordings are very effective and convenient. They are portable, readily available, and inexpensive. Be sure to use the guided audio versions provided with this book since it is not possible to actually experience yoga nidra while reading. Refer to the instructions in the Introduction to download recordings of the yoga nidra exercises in the following chapters. If you are listening in bed to help with sleep, put either a small player or just the ear buds under your pillow to keep from disturbing your sleep partner; the sound will transmit right through the pillow. If using a smartphone or similar device, put it in airplane mode to eliminate being disturbed by incoming calls and alerts, and to cut down on radio frequency energy (radio waves), a form of non-ionizing radiation.

- *Practice individually on your own.* With regular practice and because of the state of conscious awareness created during yoga nidra, it will eventually be easy to remember the content, sequence, and pacing used, especially with the help of the written instructions provided in this book. An advantage of practicing on your own is not being dependent on someone else or a recording. However, distractions are more common and you may be more likely to unintentionally fall asleep.

## Getting Ready for Yoga Nidra

Remember to keep your entire health care team informed of all the self-care measures you are doing. This includes your yoga nidra practice, exercise habits, medications, herbs, supplements and vitamins, energy work, and so on. This will aid doctors, therapists, and others in ensuring the best outcome for you. For instance, some of your medications may need to be adjusted as a result of your efforts.

## Preparing the Room for the Best Atmosphere

At first, yoga nidra is best practiced in a quiet and comfortable place where you will not be disturbed. After you get accustomed to this, practice in places that have distractions from time to time, since it is also important to get used to handling distractions. This will help you learn to keep your cool in daily living.

Consider having a designated place set aside for honoring your body, mind, and inner spirit. This can be done anywhere at home. Choose a place that provides you some personal space. It does not have to be fancy, just a place where you can have your props—blankets, bolsters, eye pillows, mat, et cetera—within reach. Add your own special touches by decorating your space for the seasons, moon cycles, or holidays—whatever appeals to you. Acknowledge your own changes and cycles, within and without. Items like pictures, mementos, candles, holy objects, and so forth can also be included to create a nice atmosphere and help you get in the mood easily and quickly. However, do not get dependent on just one place; ultimately, you should be comfortable relaxing under many different circumstances.

Here are more ways to prepare the room:

- Close the door and the windows to cut down on distractions. Shut the blinds and curtains.

- Dim the lights. If this is not possible, use night lights or carefully use candles.

- Keep the room temperature set so it is neither too warm nor too cold. Avoid being in a draft. Since your body temperature is likely to cool down when relaxing deeply, have a blanket handy in case you start feeling chilly.

- Turn off your phone and other electronic devices.

- Soft, relaxing instrumental music can enhance the environment. Play it in the background at a volume that is barely audible. This helps mask outside noises that could be distracting. Practicing in the quiet is another wonderful option.

- Let the members of your household know you are practicing yoga nidra and not to bother you until you are finished. Consider putting a "Do not disturb" sign on the door as a reminder. Move pets out of the room, too.

## Gathering Your Props for Comfort

Here are some suggested props to facilitate your experience and reduce distractions. However, don't let any of this stop you from practicing if these things are not available.

- A firm, nonslip blanket, yoga mat, beach towel, or exercise or camping mat can be used to lie on.

- A thin (one- to three-inch) cushion or pillow can support your head and maintain the neck's natural arch. Be careful: a thick pillow easily creates tension in the neck and this is to be avoided.

- An eye pillow, wash cloth, or scarf can cover your eyes. Even though your eyes will be closed, the extra darkness and weight of the eye cover enhances relaxation significantly. It calms the brain and reduces restlessness by preventing unnecessary eye movements. Do not cover your nose.

- Firm bolsters or pillows can be used to support your back and legs.

- Cover up with a cozy blanket to keep warm. Your body temperature is likely to drop during deep relaxation. Getting cold is a nuisance.

## Preparing Yourself

- Wear comfortable clothing if possible. The point is to eliminate distractions right from the start. Do not wear shoes. Socks are fine for warmth.

- Try to practice on an empty stomach. This means practicing at least a few hours after eating a heavy meal or about half an hour after a snack. Why? Your digestive system slows down during deep relaxation and it is important not to interrupt this biological process. In addition, the subtle aspects and benefits of deep relaxation are experienced and noticed more easily on an empty stomach.

- Empty your bladder.

## Getting into Position for Relaxation: Shavasana

Shavasana, known as the relaxation pose, is the yoga posture most commonly used for yoga nidra. Shavasana does not refer to the experience of yoga nidra itself. Follow these steps to get into the pose:

1. Lie down on your back on a firm surface using a yoga mat or something similar. Being on a bed or couch fosters sleep rather than yoga nidra, so lying on a clean floor is better.

2. Align yourself so there is a straight line from the center of your head, through your neck, and down to your navel.

3. Position your head so that your forehead and chin are level. Then slightly tuck your chin toward your throat. Make sure to keep the natural arch behind your neck.

4. Move your shoulders down from your ears and snuggle your shoulder blades comfortably beneath you. Place your arms along, but not touching, the sides of your body. This is the preferred position to reduce physical distractions, enhancing

relaxation. Have your palms up with fingers at ease and relaxed. This lowers sensory input from the fingertips.

5. Shift your hips and buttocks around until you feel nice and even and supported under there.

6. Place your feet about twelve to twenty-four inches apart so that the insides of your legs do not touch. Doing so relaxes the hips and back as well as cuts down on physical distractions. Let your feet rest out to each side.

7. Close your eyes or keep them slightly open.

8. Notice how all this feels and make adjustments until you feel safe and comfortable—until there is no need to move at all.

Try these adjustments, if needed:

- A rolled up towel or small pillow can aid in supporting the natural arch of the neck, if needed. Slightly elevating your head in this manner can help calm your thoughts. Plus, it can help prevent snoring if you accidently fall asleep.

- Instead of keeping your arms out to your sides, you may prefer to keep your arms closer to your body, or rest your hands over your heart or belly.

- Either use a firm pillow or bolster under your thighs or knees, or bend your knees, placing your feet flat on the floor under them, and try leaning your knees against each other. Both positions provide additional back and leg support.

- Support your entire head and back by using a rectangular yoga bolster; large, sturdy pillow; or folded nonslip blanket. With your buttocks on the floor, elevate your back, neck, and head with the bolster to a comfortable angle (try 45 degrees). Make sure that you maintain good alignment.

- See appendix 1 for optional hand positions. Called yoga mudras, they can be used to enhance respiration, reinforce your san-kalpa, and facilitate the withdrawal of the senses (*pratyahara*).

## Alternative Positions

There are always options in yoga nidra, and position is no exception.

- *Lie on your side.* Choose whichever side is most comfortable for you. Keep in mind that being on your left side can prevent heartburn, aid digestion, and may improve immunity to disease. To keep your head, neck, and spine aligned, support your head with a pillow and place another one between your knees.

- *Sit.* You can sit in a chair or on the floor as in meditation. Another way is to sit on the floor while leaning your back against a wall.

- *Stand.* Do this while leaning against a wall for support.

### When to Use Alternative Positions

- *During pregnancy:* Lie on your side, sit, or stand during preg-nancy. Do not lie on your back or stomach, especially after the first trimester.

- *To prevent snoring:* During yoga nidra, your body is in a sleep state during which you remain aware and alert. Therefore, snoring can happen. It can also happen if you accidentally fall asleep. So it's especially important to try other positions when practicing with a group of people.

- *For variety:* Use alternative positions to add variety to your practice. You can also use them to expand your ability to relax and remain alert while in different positions.

# During Your Practice

The most important thing to remember as you go into your practice is to simply follow the technique without trying to make anything happen or to obtain any particular experience or results.

**Let it be effortless.** Trying to concentrate or analyze your experience will only bog you down. Honestly, all you really have to do is listen, participate, stay aware, and welcome whatever happens with an impartial attitude.

**Remain alert and awake.** There is no harm in falling asleep during yoga nidra, but staying awake and alert is much more effective. In fact, many Yoga masters stipulate "No sleeping during yoga nidra." Here are some tips to stay awake:

- Since you will likely fall asleep if you are already tired, choose a time when you are fairly rested. In other words, rather than practicing before bedtime, practice soon after waking.

- Instead of lying on your back, try sitting in a chair or with your back against a wall. Leaning against a wall while standing is another option.

- Keep your eyes slightly open rather than closing them.

- Hold your hand up by bending at your elbow. Your hand will drop if you fall asleep, and that will awaken you.

- If you are being guided by someone, ask him or her to keep an eye on you, and give the facilitator permission to awaken you if you fall asleep.

**Stay still—or not.** Typically, we are told "no moving" during yoga nidra. Due to the deep state of relaxation experienced during yoga nidra, it will probably not even occur to you to move. In fact, it will likely feel better not to move: you'll know you could move if you wanted to, but it'll just feel better to be still. If and when you do have the urge to move, due to discomfort, restlessness, or something similar, start with witnessing the urge to move before reacting to it. First, stay still and notice what happens. The urge to move may be a temporary sensation and retreat on its own. In this case, be aware of this process unfolding. Doing this helps facilitate your understanding of the impermanent nature of things. On the other hand, if the sensation does not go away, is intolerable, or causes pain, it may need your attention. In this case, you have the option of moving—but do so mindfully rather than reactively. This principle can be applied to physical, mental, and emotional distractions as well.

**Handle distractions.** Learning to deal with distractions is important. They come in many forms, ranging from noises, stiffness, itches, coughs, and general restlessness to mentally wandering completely offtrack (thinking about grocery shopping, your to-do list, and so on). First, do your best to prevent distractions from the start with proper room setup and by preparing yourself adequately. When you notice being distracted, quickly congratulate yourself for noticing. Say something to yourself like, "Good catch." There is no need to beat yourself up or get analytical. Next, find something neutral that you feel comfortable silently saying to yourself to disengage yourself from distractions and bring your attention back to the present. Getting in the habit of using it is helpful both on and off the mat by increasing your capacity to stay alert and focused. Here are some ways to handle distractions:

- Say something like, "Oh, never mind," or "Not now, maybe later." Then gently bring your awareness back to the present.

- A passive "Oh well" is recommended by Dr. Herbert Benson and William Proctor in their *Relaxation Revolution* book (2010, 10).

- Name the distraction and let it go. Examples include "noise" or "cold" or "thought" or "planning," or whatever it happens to be.

- Rather than thinking, "I'm feeling bored and impatient," realize "Here's boredom and impatience," and explore your experience. Or say to yourself, "Isn't this interesting?" Remind yourself, "I am not my thoughts."

- Watching and waiting is very effective.

- Use mental imagery such as thinking of thoughts as weeds to be plucked and discarded, or as clouds floating by, or imagine tossing thoughts into a river to be carried away.

- Welcome the distraction with a "Hello, restless mind" or "Hello, soreness," and explore the present-moment experience. Chances are excellent that paying attention to it will lead to its disappearance. Find out for yourself.

- Play with distractions or have a conversation with them such as, "Hi, it's you again. How about going on vacation for a while," or "Bye-bye, off you go."

- Refocusing awareness on the present also works for dealing with distractions. Options to help with this include listening to whatever sounds are present; watching the designs, images, or colors as they occur on the interior of the closed eyelids; or experiencing the breath as movement or as sound. Choose whichever option works best for you, and use it until you feel centered. This is good practice for developing witness consciousness.

**Manage restlessness or racing thoughts.** A small percentage of people may experience stress instead of relaxation at first. For many, it's because they haven't noticed all the mental chattering taking place inside. Try these tips if this happens.

- Be familiar with the exercise in advance to know what to expect.

- Have a plan in place to handle restlessness or racing thoughts that is reassuring to you.

- Open your eyes for a while. Change your breathing pattern to one that comforts you.

- Be curious about your roaming thoughts rather than letting them bother you.

- Focus on something else to change the experience. For example, imagine being in a place that feels protective or calming or being surrounded by supportive people.

- Experiment to find constructive types of relaxation that do work for you.

- Try again another time, but use shorter segments.

**Understand how to treat deviations.** Deviations are different from distractions. They are a normal part of the process and often indicate progress:

- *Tuning in and out for a while is common.* It is not unusual to tune out for a while—and it's totally fine. This is when you are vaguely aware of the guiding voice in the background while still feeling relaxed and at ease. In fact, this is probably an indicator that you have entered a deeper state of relaxation on your own, so let it happen. When you notice that you have missed something, instead of trying to catch up or become critical, simply listen and follow along again. Be kind to yourself; don't judge. Just gently turn your attention back to the practice. If you no longer hear the voice, this indicates that you have fallen asleep.

- *Different segments come and go from awareness.* Folks are often surprised when they hear something "new" on the audio that they hadn't noticed before. If this happens, reassure yourself that you will hear whatever you are ready for at the right time. It is important to trust your experience, knowing that what is important for you will come to the foreground and what is irrelevant will fade into the background.

■ *Spontaneous changes start happening.* You might also notice that your experience starts becoming more spontaneous on its own. Intentionally or not, the mind starts offering its own variations to add special meaning. This is something to expect and accept, whether it happens right away or after a while. Your higher Self is actually watching out for you by providing you with what will benefit you. However, if something is disturbing, discuss it with someone you trust who has experience in these matters.

## Sequencing

The general sequence we will practice is as follows:

Part 1: Readiness and reminders (getting your room and yourself ready—proper positioning in shavasana, handling distractions, etc.)

Part 2: Setting a sankalpa

Part 3: Six stages of relaxation unfold that correspond to the *koshas* and Atma:

1. Physical (*anna maya kosha*)

2. Energetic (*prana maya kosha*)

3. Mental/emotional (*mano maya kosha*)

4. Intuitive (*vijnana maya kosha*)

5. Joy (*ananda maya kosha*)

6. Atma awareness

Part 4: Remembering the sankalpa

Part 5: Transition and return to full awareness

More specifically, the sequence used in all three yoga nidra experiences in this book follows the same basic map and progression, even if what is done during different parts changes. First, we are guided to become attentive to the here and now by becoming aware of the physical body, starting at the head. This is enhanced by paying attention to sensory input (sights, sounds, breath, feelings, and so on). Next, we move up and down the body, staying in sync with the meridians and major chakras. First on the right side, then the left, and next through the center. This particular sequence benefits the three main nerve channels (the *ida, pingala,* and *sushumna nadis*) that span from the base of the spine to the top of the head. (See "Alternate-Nostril Breathing" in appendix 2 for information on these nerve channels.) Crossing attention from one side of the body to the other is done for balancing and building neural pathways. This combined experience is relaxing, healing, and restorative.

Other valuable yoga nidra methods are available that recommend up to ten parts and a variety of formats and sequences. What is important is that they are based on the core principles of yoga nidra and are effective. Once a sequence is established, it is recommended that you stay with it to facilitate and reinforce the flow of energy (prana). You will likely find that repeating the same sequence is relaxing and comforting, and feels awkward when it is changed. N. C. Panda (2003) states in his book *Yoga-Nidra, Yogic Trance,* "The sequence should be unaltered. Maintenance of the sequence should be strictly followed" (103). He says it is okay and no harm will be done if the sequence is altered during the learning and beginning stages of practice. After a while, the sequence will be memorized and everything will be conditioned.

Richard Miller, the author of *Yoga Nidra: The Meditative Heart of Yoga* (2005) and founder of the iRest method, takes a slightly different approach. He allows for variations to the yoga nidra practice to meet the particular needs of a group or individual. For example, the usual iRest body scan begins with the mouth and follows a traditional sixty-one-point rotation of consciousness. However, when working with people experiencing sleep-related issues such as insomnia, he recommends beginning the body scan in the feet instead. In another example, when working with those who have experienced facial or pelvic trauma, these areas might initially be avoided so as not to trigger an adverse traumatic effect. The iRest practice is continually monitored, adapted, and changed as each group or person progresses in healing and learning (Miller 2015).

It is recommended that you consider these different approaches to format and sequencing to find out for yourself what works best for you.

## Transitioning Back

It is very important to consciously return to normal wakefulness with full physical, mental, and emotional awareness. This enables you to integrate the healing benefits of yoga nidra and prepares you to go on with your regular activities. For goodness' sake, it would be foolish to drive under the influence of yoga nidra!

Getting up too quickly might make you feel lightheaded. Slow it down by lying on your side for a while if you have been on your back.

Upon your return, you will most likely feel refreshed. Your mind will be very alert and you will be filled with relaxed energy. Best of all, you will be aware of your internal reservoir of peace, understanding, and joy that will continue to serve you and others.

## After Your Practice

In order to transfer the fruits of your yoga nidra practice into your daily life for stress relief, practice being aware of the signals that your body, mind, and emotions give you throughout the day. Learn to relax the tension in your neck and shoulders *before* you get that stress-induced headache.

Take yoga and mindfulness breaks throughout the day to remain relaxed and empowered. For instance, use your breath for bringing yourself into moment-to-moment awareness, soothing your nerves, calming your restless mind, and refreshing your energy. (Refer to appendices 2 and 3 for more options.)

Practice remembering and reliving your new relaxation and awareness skills. Once you start feeling the short- and long-term results, you will be eager to practice more often.

## Design a Practice Plan That Is Right for You

There is no better time than now to design a yoga nidra practice that will meet your needs. Start by thinking about how to approach this using the recommendations below. Use your journal to put your action plan in writing.

**Dedicate time to your practice.** Decide on a time of day or night that works for you and your household. This could be upon getting up in the morning (perfect for morning people), during the midday, or perhaps at the close of the day. Routine helps. Do your best to stay with the time you choose. *Use your journal to write down what time frame you will follow.*

**Set realistic goals.** Decide to practice for a reasonable amount of time daily so as not to get discouraged. The time is variable; the most important thing is that you set some time aside for your practice. Perhaps start by committing to practice the parts of yoga nidra most valuable to you for five to fifteen minutes per day and build from there. Any practice, even one that seems restless or of little value, is better than no practice. *Write down how much time you will give to yourself.*

**Create a special place for yoga nidra.** It will be easier to practice if you have a place for it. Set it up as soon as possible. *Jot some notes down on where your special place will be and the things you will have in it.*

**Look at your lifestyle choices.** Perhaps it is time to make some changes in support of your health and yoga nidra practice. Make sure you are getting enough sleep, proper nutrition, and adequate exercise. Are there other lifestyle habits that need to be broken or established? For instance, it will be difficult to feel calm and peaceful if you ingest too much caffeine. *Write down your notes on improving your lifestyle in your journal.*

**Use your journal.** Record the date and the amount of time spent practicing. Include notes on what you experienced. Insights are often fleeting and forgotten, so writing them down will help. Looking over your notebook from time to time will show you the progress being made.

**Register for a yoga nidra course or start a practice group of your own.** Practicing with other people is motivating and will help you establish a consistent practice.

## Overcoming Excuses

Even with all the benefits of yoga nidra, people are still hesitant to practice. Unfortunately, misunderstandings still exist. Let's clear up some of these common myths:

**"I'm not the type."** Much of contemporary yoga has misled people into thinking it is for a specific type of person. In reality, yoga is valuable for everybody, no matter the age, fitness level, health status, nationality, economic status, gender, tradition, or faith.

**"I'm not flexible."** All that is required for yoga nidra is lying down, therefore flexibility is not needed. Patanjali's Yoga Sutra II.46 advises being steady and comfortable.

**"I can't afford it."** All that is needed is a comfortable place to practice along with understanding yoga's essential principles and practices. There is no need to enroll in a class (though classes have some advantages). This book and the downloadable audio recordings are plenty to get you started, help you gain the full benefits of yoga nidra, and support a lifelong practice.

**"I don't like classes or groups"** or **"I don't have the discipline to practice on my own."** All types of yoga can be practiced in either a group setting or alone as a personal practice. Since both approaches have their advantages and disadvantages, choose what works the best for you. Keep in mind that practicing with a guided audio file can be an excellent middle ground.

**"It's against my religion"** or **"I'm not religious."** Yoga is not a religion unto itself. Yoga masters will encourage you to practice your own religion, if you have one, and are not interested in changing it. Yoga's wisdom teachings encourage people to follow the religious or spiritual path of their upbringing or of their own choice. Encouragement is given to study scriptures for guidance and inspiration (*svadhyaya*), and specific scriptures are not held up over others. The Vedas, one of the oldest wisdom texts of Yoga, tells us that "Truth is one, paths are many." This is respectful and inclusive of different beliefs, cultures, and faith traditions. During my many years of teaching, scores of people have shared with me that yoga has deepened their own faith. I remember one woman who left her successful business to go to divinity school and became a Christian minister, all fueled by her yoga practice.

# What to Remember

- You cannot go wrong when practing yoga nidra. All that is needed is to listen, participate, and stay alert. In fact, whatever is experienced is to be explored and accepted. You are in charge of your experience. The teachings and practices in this book will lead the way.

- A sankalpa adds depth to your yoga nidra practice.

- Prepare your setting and yourself properly.

- Yoga nidra is a complete practice in and of itself. Regular practice builds on itself, and the benefits are cumulative. While regular practice is ideal, some practice is better than no practice.

- Support your health and yoga nidra practice with healthy lifestyle choices.

- Lean toward confidence.

## Chapter 4

# Relax: Deep Relaxation for Unshakable Peace and Inner Joy

Your understanding of how yoga nidra solves stress while promoting physical health, peace of mind, and an awakened spirit is in place. In addition, your foundations are also in order.

Now is the time to put this new information and your new skills into practice, and practice is what it takes. Just like learning any new skill, practice and repetition is necessary to become competent and to reap the full benefits of yoga nidra and its components. No one would expect a flute player to be able to play musically after only a few lessons—it takes time and attention to learn the fingerings, get a few notes to play, and read the music. The same goes for sports as well as hobbies—your favorite sports professional has spent years perfecting his or her game, and the same will be true for relaxation training. In the beginning, you might fall asleep instead of experiencing real relaxation and yoga nidra. Only one or two levels of relaxation may be experienced rather than all five of them, or it might be hard to lie still for very long. Even so, you will benefit immensely. Therefore, there is no need to be in a hurry; in fact, that approach will only slow you down and spoil the fun.

A yoga nidra student once said, "Yoga nidra is such a luscious treat to be savored. It's the dark chocolate of yoga."

## Relaxing Journey Through the Koshas

This first yoga nidra experience is a journey through the *koshas*, the layers that surround and cover your peaceful, joyful, enduring Self, as described in chapter 2. Taking time to systematically relax each of these layers and to return your attention to full awareness is essential for complete stress relief. It enables you to integrate all these levels of yourself and can clear your mind, reduce pain and suffering, and give you a felt sense of well-being, bringing you to a place of understanding, unconditional joy, deep restfulness, and restoration. Here is a further understanding of the technique used for each of the koshas.

## Relaxing and Restoring the Physical Body (Anna Maya Kosha)

It is vital to be able to recognize physical tightness and holding patterns, as well as to have reliable methods for reducing physical tension brought on by stress. Physical tension contributes to soreness, fatigue, poor circulation, and pain. This makes it very important to learn what physical tension feels like as well as how physical relaxation feels, enabling you to recognize tension before a bit of tightness in your neck and shoulders, for instance, becomes a full-blown headache. You will soon know how to replace too much tightness with just the right amount of effort needed. Relaxation is actually experiential and not merely a technique, thought, or plan.

In this yoga nidra practice, progressive muscle relaxation is used for inducing physical relaxation. This technique was first developed in the early 1920s and taught by Edmund Jacobson, an American physician. During it, each muscle group is systemically and intentionally tensed and then released. Fighting tension with tension is like fighting fire with fire. It does not seem like it would work, but it does.

Your energy begins to flow again once it is not being stopped up with tension and stress. Think of a garden hose. If there is a kink in the hose, the water stops and will not flow. When the kink is released, the water can move once again. The same principle applies to muscular tension. Once the tension and blocked energy is released, your vitality will spring back to life and can be used in useful and meaningful ways.

# Introduction to Progressive Muscle Relaxation

Let's try this powerful technique right now.

First, notice how your face feels in this moment. Determine where there is tension and relaxation. Are you gritting your teeth? Do you feel a soft smoothness around your eyes? What else do you notice? Rate it on a scale of one to ten: The lower end of the scale indicates feelings of relaxation, and lacking muscular tightness and holding. The higher end of the scale reflects a great deal of holding and pressure. What number reflects your overall level of facial tension? Write it here: _____.

Now, bring your attention to your eyebrows. Lift your eyebrows up toward your hairline for a few moments and then let them release. This time, lower your eyebrows toward your chin, hold temporarily, and then relax. Now, scrunch and squeeze your eyes shut and then let the tension go. Allow any remaining tension to smooth away. Notice any difference in the area around your eyes.

Next, bring your attention to your mouth. How does it feel right now? Begin pursing your lips tightly together, followed by totally relaxing and releasing the tension. Press your tongue against the roof of your mouth and let it go. Gently move your jaw up and down, sideways, and all around. Now, let your jaw rest and relax, allowing your teeth to part slightly and softening the corners of your lips. You are invited to take a big breath in through your nose and to sigh it out a few times.

Once again, notice how your face feels. Do you have more awareness in your face now? Can you feel how tightness and tension has decreased? Does your face feel more at ease? What else do you notice? Rate it from one to ten. Write it here: _____.

As you can see, stress relief can be done quickly, easily, and in the moment; it does not have to be long and complicated. This technique can be used at any time and can be applied to any area of your body, day or night.

We will soon use this technique throughout your entire body. After bringing awareness to your head and face, we will start tensing and releasing every muscle group in the body. The sequence to be used is based on the mindbody connection. The brain is divided into left and right hemispheres that are connected by the *corpus callosum*. The left hemisphere of the brain primarily dominates the right side of the body and vice versa. This is evident when someone suffers a stroke on the right side of the brain and it impacts the left side of the body. Even though the hemispheres work together, each hemisphere has different tendencies and functions. In general, the left hemisphere tends to have a greater influence on the logical, rational thought processes. The right side favors abstract, intuitive, and subjective thought patterns. In theory, the restless mind will begin calming down if we start on the right side of the body since it influences the functioning of the left hemisphere of the brain. This is also in keeping with the *ida* and *pingala nadis* (nerve channels) as described by yogis and outlined in appendix 2.

When physical tension releases, you will notice that your body feels heavy, like you are sinking into whatever you are sitting or lying on. This is a good sign, so let it happen. It is the first stage of relaxation.

## Relaxing Energetically
## (Prana Maya Kosha)

After relaxing physically, we will next turn our attention to the energy body, or layer. This subtle and powerful life force activates our physicality and is primarily accessed through breathing. The mind and breath govern and mirror each other. Have you ever noticed how easy it is to hold your breath when you are on edge? How about how shallow or arrhythmic the breath gets when you are under stress? When you pay attention, you will notice how your breathing becomes full and easy when you are relaxing in your favorite easy chair and surrounded by whatever brings you genuine comfort. This sense of relaxed energy can be carried over into daily living.

During this stage of relaxation, a sense of deep stillness is noticed along with the relaxed, heavy feeling. This is the second stage of relaxation.

To accomplish this, we will go through the entire body again. This time, we will use the breath consciously while focusing on each part of the body as in the previous segment. This time, however, you will be guided to intentionally take a nice, big breath in while becoming aware of each muscle group and breathing out any tension, discomfort, or tightness with the exhalation.

As Nischala Joy Devi explains so well in *The Healing Path of Yoga*, "When we are able to balance the energy *in* our legs, we are able to balance the energy on our legs and that physical balance gives us stability in everything we do" (2000, 70).

## Mental and Emotional Relaxation (Mano Maya Kosha)

We all have experienced how our thoughts, emotions, and feelings can bring on the stress. Have you ever been physically exhausted but cannot seem to get any rest or fall into a sound sleep because your mind keeps racing?

It is all too easy to ruin a perfectly fine time by being mentally distracted rather than to experience the present moment. How often have you let yourself get upset by rehashing regrets from the past or by worrying about the future? In addition, the body can serve as a holding tank for thoughts and emotions that have been ignored or repressed.

This third stage of relaxation can help heal these scars and free up your mental energy to boot. It can clear out the debris and bring about a keen state of awareness without unnecessary thinking or mental effort.

By now, your body is so thoroughly relaxed that it only requires a small amount of breath. That breath will naturally be soft, quiet, and subtle. Your exhalation will automatically lengthen and your chest will hardly move while breathing.

This subtle breath is used throughout the body to mentally "brush and sweep away" current thoughts and sensations, lingering memories, and remnants of old injuries. Analysis is not needed here. That would be like sifting and sorting through the trash before throwing it out.

This level of relaxation brings about the sensation of feeling light. This is because you are not being "held down" by physical and energetic stresses. Thoughts can naturally rise to the surface and become released.

## Relaxing into Intuition
## (Vijnana Maya Kosha)

Our inbuilt intuition and higher intellect is revealed during the fourth stage of relaxation. This aspect is automatically accessed without the distraction of physical and energetic stress, and from the natural release of thoughts, feelings, and memories. During this period, it is common to feel a further sense of lightness. It can even feel like you are floating. Buoyant. Weightless. In addition, there is a sense of detach-ment present. We are in a place of feeling peace and contentment, independent of having to have things be anything other than what they are, or needing anything to "go just right." What a treasure when this attitude carries over into daily living.

During this period, the breath is very still and quiet. All that is needed in this stage is to observe a minute or so of this complete solitude.

A nonmental state of being is experienced that opens us up to our source of higher knowledge and wisdom. Insights are often revealed. Answers to your questions may be discovered. Wisdom is uncovered.

## Experiencing Unshakable Peace and Joy
## (Ananda Maya Kosha)

The fifth stage of yoga nidra is indescribable because it actually goes beyond words and way beyond the thinking mind into pure con-tentment. What is experienced is total relaxation along with a pro-found sense of inner and outer stillness. It feels very peaceful and quiet.

Timeless. It is referred to as the "body of joy" and is downright blissful.

You will be invited to open yourself to this deeply relaxing state and will remain there for a few more minutes.

## Atma Awareness

Experiencing the Atma often happens naturally in the sixth stage of yoga nidra.

## The Return

The process of coming back to full alertness is as important as the process was in getting there. Coming out slowly and purposefully will enable a profound integration to take place for the body, mind, and spirit.

Before coming back, however, you will be given the opportunity to remember and reinforce your intention (*sankalpa*). In time, whatever you plant in this rich and fertile soil of your being will become a reality because you will have transcended the conscious mind.

During this period of returning, the reverse order is used when bringing your attention back to full awareness.

## Skill Building: Yoga Nidra for Unshakable Peace and Joy

To get the full benefits of yoga nidra, an audio version of the following exercise is available for download (visit http://www.newharbinger .com/31823, or see the instructions in the Introduction). Feel free to familiarize yourself with the process by reading through the entire script first. Note that, for this and all the scripts in this book, ellipses (…) and the spaces between paragraphs indicate that you should take a brief pause. When you see "[Pause]," wait a little longer. Before listening to the audio for this practice, review the reminders given in chapter 3 for getting the most out of your yoga nidra experience. In time, you will be able to guide yourself from memory. If you are leading someone else through this exercise, please refer to the tips for doing so in appendix 4.

## Part 1: Readiness and Reminders

Choose a place where you'll feel comfortable and are unlikely to be disturbed. Get your props ready, shut the door, dim the lights, and turn off the phone or whatever else might be distracting.

### Relaxation Pose (Shavasana)

Stretch yourself out on a thick blanket or mat on the floor. Either close your eyes or keep them slightly open... To help you relax your hips and legs, try letting your heels be about two feet apart. It's fine to make your own adjustments so that your legs and hips feel comfortable and at ease... Allow your feet and toes to rest out to the sides, and let go... Now, bring your attention to your hips... Notice how the weight of your hips is resting on the ground... If it feels uneven, lift them up slightly, then settle back down until it feels even and balanced on both sides.

Shift your attention to your shoulders. Feel the placement of your shoulders, exactly where they are... You're invited to move your shoulders down from your ears and tuck your shoulder blades under for more support. Have your arms out to each side with your palms up.

Settle the very back of your head on the floor or thin cushion and tuck your chin so that it's slightly lower than your forehead. Adjust your hair if it's in the way. Make sure that your head and neck are nicely aligned with your spine.

Feel free to adjust your clothing and props, making sure that every part of your body feels as steady and comfortable as possible.

Remind yourself to let the yoga nidra process happen naturally by being openly aware. It's common to tune out while feeling deeply quiet and at ease while vaguely aware of what's happening outside. Return your attention to the guiding instructions if you get distracted unnecessarily. Go ahead and add your own personal reminders for keeping on track and having a more meaningful time. Say it positively and in the present tense.

Please take a big breath in through your nose and sigh it out through your mouth… Feel free to breathe in and sigh out a few more times.

## Part 2: Setting a Sankalpa

Setting a sankalpa, a personal resolve, enhances your yoga nidra experience immensely and helps transfer the benefits received into daily life. It's a statement that conveys a positive trait to deeply benefit you in living your life in a more healthy and meaningful way.

You may use this time to formulate one that has meaning for you, letting it come to you. Tune in with your heart and soul for the one that lights you up and ignites your energy. Keep it simple, positive, and brief. Use the present tense as if it's already happened… If you have one, remember it now and begin clearly and sincerely stating it a few times. Be consistent, keeping the same one over time.

[Pause]

Sense what it would be like if it were already true. How would things be different?

[Pause]

Take a big breath in…and let it go.

# Part 3: Yoga Nidra in Six Stages

## Stage 1: *Progressive Muscle Relaxation for Physical Relaxation (Anna Maya Kosha)*

Now, bring your awareness to your breathing, just as it is... In your own way, remind yourself to stay awake and alert, even when you're resting and relaxing very deeply. It's time to relax physically by letting go of muscular tension.

### Head and Face

Let's start with your head. Begin to notice where the back of your head touches the surface it's on. Feel the very place of contact. Let your head become more and more supported by allowing it to rest into the support that is present for you.

Now, become aware of your face... All at once, start squeezing your eyes and forehead, scrunch up your nose and cheeks, and bring tension to your lips and mouth. Holding it for a second or two...and completely let go... Letting all the muscles soften...more and more. Allowing your forehead to smooth out...your eyes to rest and become still...even your eyelids...and especially at the corners. Letting relaxation now comfort your nose and cheeks...and letting go, even more, of any tension around your mouth. If you wish, allow your teeth and lips to part slightly...letting your tongue rest softly in your mouth... and allowing the corners of your lips to completely let go. There's no need for a facial expression of any type. Simply let your whole face soften and relax, more and more, melting with relaxation.

### Right Arm

And now, bring your awareness to your right arm, become aware of your arm from your hand on up to your shoulder...and now tighten your hand into a fist...and move the tension up your arm to your shoulder…and now open your fingers up wide…and all at once, let go of all the squeezing and tension…allowing the muscles to relax…staying aware of the changing feelings and sensations as they come and go.

This process of tensing and releasing shows you how tension and relaxation actually feel. These skills are very useful to have.

## Right Leg

Now, bring your awareness to your right leg, from your foot on up to your hip, and begin to tense up the muscles, just squeezing the muscles…and feel the tension…and now, all at once, relax, letting all the tension drain away… Feel the muscles relaxing…feeling heavy and relaxed.

And now, letting go into the heaviness and comfort of relaxation.

## Left Arm

Shift your awareness over to your left hand and make a tight fist and feel the tension go into your arm and up to your shoulder… spread your fingers out wide…and finally, totally letting go…feeling the heaviness and comfort of relaxation spreading through your shoulders, arms, and hands.

Feel free to clear your throat and, if needed, to change your position.

## Left Leg

Bring your awareness to your left leg, from your foot on up to your hip… Begin to squeeze the muscles up to the bones…feel the squeeze…and now, let go totally…let go, allowing your entire leg to relax and noticing a comfortable heaviness in both of your legs as they relax more and more.

Notice how your mind can be alert, even as your body continues relaxing more and more... You may be noticing the feelings of relaxation being experienced as heaviness. This is the feeling of muscles relaxing, so let it happen. Let yourself remain alert while you're relaxing, more and more, observing what relaxation feels like.

## Trunk

Bring your awareness to your buttocks and squeeze these muscles and feel the tension...and now relax, feeling tension melting safely away...allowing all the tightness and tension to drain away from around your hips.

If you would prefer, you may put your feet on the floor with your knees above them.

Begin pressing your naval inward and feel the tension...pressing the naval in...and now relax and soften the naval area...relaxing and softening, more and more... This time push your abdomen outward and feel the abdominal wall stretch, making some room inside, and hold... Now relax...softening the muscles more and more, feeling the relief... And each time you softly breathe out, you can relax even more, letting go of more tension.

## Neck, Face, and Head

Bring your awareness to your neck and throat. You're invited to softly and gently roll your head from side to side...and to bring it back to rest.

Bring your awareness to your jaw, and open your mouth and move your jaw all around, letting go of tension in your jaw...and now relax and become still...letting your teeth part slightly...relaxing the corners of your lips... You can even moisten your lips if you'd like... And now, press your tongue against the roof of your mouth or to the back of your teeth...and let go...relaxing your tongue, and resting it comfortably in your mouth... Notice the moisture in your mouth... Experience the moisture...and all the space that's inside.

And even though your eyes are closed, squeeze your eyes...and your forehead, feeling the constriction...and letting go...and your forehead releases and smoothes out like silk.

Feel your body resting deeply...feeling more content and comforted by the relaxation...simply experiencing the deep heaviness of relaxation.

Just for a moment, you may barely open your eyes if you wish...and let them close...feel the relief... Can you feel where your eyelids touch?

## Stage 2: Energy Body Awareness (Prana Maya Kosha)

If you would like to relax further now, you can...just become more and more aware of your breathing...simply noticing your breathing as it comes and goes. This will relax you energetically.

Please remember, this is a time to consciously and mindfully relax and not for sleeping. So, in your own way, remind yourself to stay alert.

Once again, take your awareness to your head and face... Without moving, take in a big intentional breath and let it go, feeling your face relaxing even more. All around your forehead...releasing even more around your eyes...your nose and cheeks...and now, allow your mouth to relax...softening both inside and on the outside.

Guide your awareness to your arms. Without moving your arms, take a big conscious breath in and let it go, feeling your arms rest and relax, more and more. Allowing your arms to become quite still.

Become aware of your legs... Without moving your legs, take a conscious breath in...and breathe out, and feel your legs relax even more.

Notice the presence of deep stillness...Knowing you could move if you really wanted or needed to, but it just feels so much better not moving.

And now, bring your awareness to your hips...mindfully breathing in, become more aware of your hips...and when breathing out, relaxing your hips even more...letting go with each and every exhalation...feeling the heaviness and stillness of relaxing.

And now, bring your awareness to your belly... Take a deep breath in...and breathe out, letting go of all tension in and around your belly.

Bring your awareness around your heart and lungs and take in a big, full breath...a little more...and exhaling completely, your chest settles comfortably into relaxation... And yet your mind is alert and aware of what's happening...breathing and allowing your awareness to rest all around your heart.

Letting all of the muscles relax...and the body relaxes totally... noticing how comfortable and heavy you feel...feeling a blanket of relaxation surrounding you with quietness and calmness. Just let it happen...being aware of how relaxation feels.

Notice what you're experiencing right here and now.

[Pause]

If you'd like, feel free to shift around a little or adjust your clothes or props.

## Stage 3: Relaxing Mental and Emotional Stress
## (Mano Maya Kosha)

And now, notice how soft and quiet and subtle your breath has become... Leave it alone and let it be...just allowing your breathing to be soft and subtle, so gentle that your chest hardly moves. It's okay, not much breath is needed now.

Perhaps you'd like to go further still into relaxation for some mental and emotional relief... If you would, use your natural breath like a broom to begin sweeping away thoughts and beliefs, feelings and memories, just for now, from your face and head...sweeping and brushing tensions away from your face and head. Easily and smoothly, sweeping, and brushing stress away, whether past or present. Repairing and healing and restoring.

Bring your attention back to your arms and let your breath naturally begin sweeping down your arms to your hands now...removing thoughts and feelings and memories. Even pain and old injuries. Brushing and sweeping and rinsing away.

As this is done, you may notice the heaviness being replaced with feelings of being lightweight...and lighter still.

Bring your attention down to your legs and feet, and let your breath be like a sweeping motion, sweeping down your legs and feet with your breath, erasing thoughts, rinsing away memories and feelings...hurts vanishing...brushing tension away with your soft and subtle breath...removing thoughts and memories...and any old injuries are swept clean with your breath as it flows down your legs to your feet and safely away.

And having your awareness around your hips and with your soft subtle breath, sweep tensions away, allowing your breath to release old pain…sweeping stress away, and allowing relaxation to happen, more and more. Healing and restoring.

And as relaxation deepens, it may feel as if you're floating…let this happen. Feeling buoyant.

And feel the sweeping and brushing and rinsing breath in and around the vital organs of your abdomen…softening and lightening…releasing tension and old, forgotten hurts…removing any remaining tension, wiping away old pains and injuries with your subtle breath in around your vital organs…and it lessens and lightens with the soft and subtle breath.

And now this sweeping motion moves all around your chest and heart…and memories and hurts are swept away, injuries and tensions are cleared out with your gentle breath…nice and clean. Sweeping and brushing away outdated feelings and emotions. Repairing and healing and restoring all around your chest and heart.

Feeling quite peaceful, use this technique around your neck and throat…rinsing away unspoken words…clearing…and as the tensions release, the connection between your head and heart opens and becomes free and clear and easy…simply brushing with your gentle breath.

And now sweeping and smoothing around your ears…softening more and more…brushing away hurtful sounds of any type, like harmful things you may have been told…and as this clearing continues, your sense of inner hearing is awakened.

And now your breath brushes all around your eyes, removing visions that are no longer helpful…and your inner eyes open…and your inner vision clears.

And let any last, little bit of tension disappear through the top of the head.

Observe the buoyancy...the softness...even the weightlessness of deep relaxation...it's like a detached feeling from the body, and the mind...and being detached from worldly cares, just for now.

[Pause, one minute]

### Stage 4: Relaxing into Intuition (Vijnana Maya Kosha)

And if you like, you can go further and deeper still by discovering and finding a place, sensing a place inside where your inner knowing is alive and well... It's a place of awareness where the insights and wisdom you've been searching for can find you now. During this quiet time, let yourself be open and receptive to receive whatever will serve your highest good.

[Pause for one to two minutes]

### Stage 5: Experiencing Unshakable Peace and Joy (Ananda Maya Kosha)

And if you wish, you can go further and deeper still by finding a place, sensing a place where inner joy dwells...a place to rest in stillness and tranquility...a place to experience unshakable wholeness and connection and completeness...and your awareness is open and very still during this time of quiet.

[Pause for two to three minutes]

### Stage 6: Atma for Dwelling in One's True Self

Let this all go for now into the quiet, residing in awareness, dwelling peacefully here and now, allowing awareness of your true Self to be Present.

[Pause two to four minutes]

## Part 4: Remembering Your Sankalpa

Om shanti—peace, peace, peace... Now review and remember your sankalpa. Bring your sankalpa back to mind. Repeat the same sankalpa made at the beginning. Say it with your heart several times, planting it deep inside and becoming even more rooted and growing.

[Pause one to two minutes]

## Part 5: Transition Back to Full Awareness

It's time to start making the transition back... Without having to move in any way, bring your awareness back to the breath...and simply follow the breath with your awareness through your body. Awakening with each breath.

Bringing your awareness to the center of your heart and to your breathing...becoming more and more aware of your body.

Bring your awareness to the top of your head and feel your head and face awaken...your sense of vision... And listening and hearing awakens as you become more and more aware, listening to the sounds in the room.

And now your attention flows through your neck and throat, and, if you'd like, slowly roll your head from side to side, feeling the movement...and let yourself become still again.

And your awareness flows through your spine and to your arms and legs.

When you're ready, begin stretching all over, more and more... moving and waking up your body and mind, heart and soul.

It's time to come back into full awareness and wakefulness and bring back with you all the benefits of yoga nidra to help yourself as well as to benefit others.

When you're ready, roll over onto your side, and curl up.

[Pause]

To come up to sitting, press your hands and arms down to lift yourself up to sitting... Touch the tips of your thumbs to the tips of your index fingers and rest your hands on your knees to seal it in.

Allow your eyes to close again, and relish the inner stillness...the peace and joy... Open your eyes up just a sliver...notice more light...and close them again and rest... Slowly blink your eyes open and closed to blend the inner world with the outer world... move and stretch if you like, and when your eyes completely open, you'll feel Present, alert, and relaxed.

## Variations

To start, it is highly recommended that you become familiar with and practice the entire exercise. This will enable you to become comfortable with the sequence and the whole experience of yoga nidra fully. Best of all, you will gain relief from physical, energetic, mental, and emotional stress and uncover the unshakable peace and joy that is always present. Once this is realized, you will be able to feel calm in the midst of whatever is swirling around you.

After you are comfortable with the entire exercise, you may want to try out these recommendations and variations:

■ *Always begin and end with your sankalpa.* Doing so will help you keep your focus during the exercise. Having and using a sankalpa will make it possible for real changes to occur for you. Yoga nidra takes you to a brain wave state where this happens.

- *Try different body positions.* Rather than lying down on your back, practice yoga nidra while on your side. Another option is to practice yoga nidra while sitting or even standing while leaning against a wall.

- *Try different hand positions.* Rather than having your hands out to each side with your palms up, use the *kubera mudra* while setting and remembering your sankalpa, to enhance its effectiveness. Refer to appendix 1 for instructions on how to use mudras.

- *Vary the amount of physical tension used during stage 1.* For instance, instead of tensing each muscle group to the maximum amount, try tensing only 50 percent of the way. Other times, only use a level of tension that can just be noticed.

- *Pair the body parts.* After you are accustomed to going through each area of the body individually, you can begin to do both arms at the same time, both legs at the same time, and so on.

- *Simplify the practice.* Another option is to practice only relaxing progressively throughout the body or to concentrate only on the breathing awareness.

- *Use different sequences.* For example, instead of starting with the head and then going through the right arm and leg, then the left arm and leg, et cetera, start with the right leg, then the left leg, right arm, left arm, et cetera. Another option is to start at your feet and work up to your head. Just do not leave anything out. Find the sequence that works best for you and then keep it as your foundation by using it again and again. Repeating the same sequence will energetically ingrain the process for you. After a while, it is fine to change the sequence for variety occasionally.

# What to Remember

■ Remember to use the audio download provided with this book.

■ Yoga nidra progresses in stages of relaxation. Take your time to develop your relaxation skills and enjoy the journey.

■ In the beginning, you may only experience a few stages or fall asleep. This is fine. You will still benefit immensely. With practice and intention, you will eventually have the complete experience of yoga nidra—conscious deep sleep.

■ Consistent practice is needed for lasting results.

■ Lean toward beauty and grace.

## Chapter 5

# Reflect: Yoga Nidra for Sensing Inner Strength and Balance

L et's explore and practice another remarkable way to experience yoga nidra. It can be used as a great remedy for counteracting physical tension and the limiting beliefs and feelings identified during the Assess Your Stress questionnaire in chapter 1. Profound relaxation for healing, inner balance, and peace are cultivated.

"Exhilarating!" is how Jeanne described her first experience with yoga nidra. She said, "It truly raised my spirit. I felt so relaxed, as if in a state of euphoria. It's a wonderful meditation. While in this state, there were no physical or mental thoughts. Just oneness… I never experienced such a depth of meditation in my fifteen years of daily practice as a nun."

The mindbody tools used for this next yoga nidra experience involve the progression through the layers of *koshas* using a sensory awareness and body scan technique, a breathing meditation, and guided imagery. As always, a *sankalpa* will be used at the beginning and end of the practice. To deepen your experience, it is important to have an understanding of these tools and concepts and how it all works.

## Sensory Awareness and Body Scanning for the Physical Stage (Anna Maya Kosha)

Physical relaxation begins with practicing sensory awareness, with special attention being paid to sight, touch, and sound. This brings your focus to the here and now and away from thoughts based on the past or future.

Using the sense of sight is a very effective centering technique, because vision only occurs moment-to-moment. Have you ever noticed that you can still see even with your eyes closed? All that is needed is to try. Darkness, designs, colors, spots, or a combination are possibilities of what can be seen when paying attention. What you see does not matter. What matters is passively focusing your attention on what is being seen and watching it as it changes. Have fun watching whatever appears as it comes and goes on the inside screen of your closed eyelids. This brings you into the moment and quickly settles down mental restlessness. Yogis refer to watching this inner space of consciousness as *chidakasha.*

Time is also spent listening to various sounds as they come and go. Naming the sounds or preferring some and resisting others gets in the way and is to be avoided. When you notice this happening, just go back to simply listening. The thinking mind quickly settles down and restlessness is transformed into relaxation.

## Understanding the Sensory-Motor Cortex

The next stage revolves around scanning your body mentally. Have you ever watched a documentary demonstrating what happens when a person's brain matter is carefully stimulated with probes? What happens is that physical movements and feelings occur as a result of the probing. For instance, one area being probed causes a physical movement somewhere in the body, whereas another might bring on laughter or tears. This is an expression of the brain-body connection. Yoga's Ayurvedic healers figured this out ages ago, but instead of stimulating the brain with probes to cause a bodily reaction, the opposite was done. They brilliantly realized that mentally scanning the body in a particular way affects the brain positively. The nerve pathways between the body and brain become clear and are strengthened, facilitating deeply healing relaxation.

The order and duration used during this mental scanning is based on the areas of the body corresponding to the brain's sensory-motor cortex, also called the *homunculus*. If you look closely at the diagram, you will notice that more area in this part of the brain is devoted to certain places than to others. For instance, compare the relatively large amount of space dedicated to the hands and fingers with the small amount dedicated to the hips. This is why more time is intentionally spent scanning the areas of the body with more of the brain dedicated to it during the practice.

To replace restless thoughts with peace of mind, the scan moves at a pace that gives enough time to experience each spot but not enough time to think about it. This has the potential to enhance self-esteem by replacing poor or outdated opinions of your body and mind with impartiality and detachment. Furthermore, mentally moving back and forth between the right and left sides of the body during another portion of the mental scanning further enhances brain hemisphere and body integration.

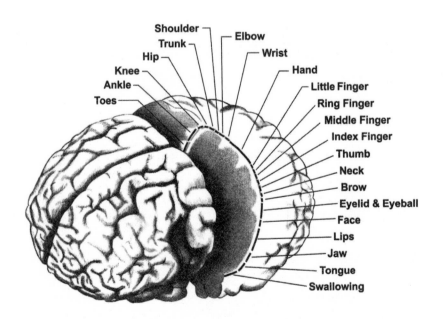

# Breath and Chakra Awareness for the Energetic Stage (Prana Maya Kosha)

A breathing meditation is used for the prana maya kosha. During this stage, you will consciously and mindfully follow the natural breath, bringing your attention back to it each time your mind wanders. This calms the nervous system and develops concentration, patience, and self-compassion.

## Understanding the Chakras

The next diagram shows the primary energetic centers that are also scanned mentally. These centers, called chakras, are described as spinning wheels of subtle energy and are located at places from the base of the spine to the crown of the head. Chakras influence the health of every system of the body and are an important indicator of a person's well-being. Each chakra has its own value and importance rather than one taking precedence over another. They can have excessive or deficient energy, which can have a harmful effect on overall health. Furthermore, they guide and govern the developmental stages of our body, mind, and emotions, and progressively awaken our potential as spiritual beings. Chakras are said to house the universal energy of life (prana) and one's guiding intelligence (Lusk 2005a, 2005b). Scanning the chakras during the first stage of yoga nidra can support healing and rejuvenation, and it serves as an effective segue into working with the energetic body (prana maya kosha) and our mental/emotional nature (mano maya kosha), as well as in subsequent stages.

The following illustration indicates the location and identity of the major chakras, along with a brief summary of what happens when they are healthy and balanced, as well as the lessons and challenges of each. The chakras are not actual physical structures within the body; rather, they are energetic in nature. But just because they cannot be seen does not mean they do not exist. The wind is invisible but it can still be felt; it is an important element and can have a range of effects on the environment. The same is true of the chakras.

Compare these characteristics with what you marked on the Assess Your Stress questionnaire in chapter 1. The guided imagery portion of this practice focuses on balancing these areas and concepts.

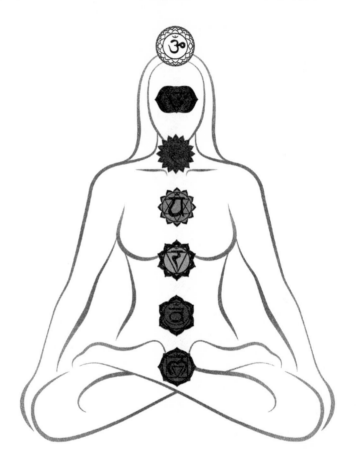

*Crown chakra:* This chakra is located at the top of the head and identifies with the universal. It connects you with your sacred wisdom source without intellectualizing or being rigid in your thinking and attitudes. Its lesson is about Self-knowledge and its challenge is attachment. Its primary color is violet.

*Third-eye chakra:* The next chakra is located between and just above the eyebrows. It identifies with the archetypal. It is involved in becoming intuitive and learning to trust your instincts instead of relying too heavily on authorities or living in a fantasy world. Its lesson is self-reflection and its challenge is illusion. Its primary color is indigo.

*Throat chakra:* This chakra is at the throat and is identified with the creative. It is related to your ability to express yourself and listen accurately. It helps you know when and how to speak truthfully and when to be quiet. Its lesson is about self-expression and its challenge is deceit. Its primary color is light blue.

*Heart chakra:* The middle chakra has a relational identity. It is linked to having compassion and kindness for yourself and others. The heart chakra helps you have harmonious relationships without being over-bearing or shy. Its lesson is self-acceptance and its challenge is grief. Its primary color is a spring green.

*Solar plexus chakra:* Located between the heart and upper abdomen, this chakra is identified with the ego. When balanced, it is correlated with having good self-esteem and being decisive instead of being timid or domineering. Its lesson is self-definition and its challenge is shame. Its primary color is yellow.

*Sacral chakra:* This chakra is in the pelvic area and its identity is emotional. It is associated with the ability to express healthy feelings, creativity, and intimacy without being overly attached or distant to others. Its lesson is self-gratification and its challenge is guilt. Its primary color is orange.

*Root chakra:* Located at the base of the spine, the root chakra's identity is physical. It governs the ability to feel secure, grounded, and stable without being materialistic, greedy, or obsessed. Its lesson is self-preservation and its challenge is fear. Its primary color is red.

More than 100 *marma points* were identified by Ayurvedic yogis long ago. A marma point, each with its own intelligence and consciousness, is where flesh, veins, arteries, tendons, bones, and joints meet up anatomically. These vital points are also closely connected to thoughts, perceptions, and emotions, and are believed to provide an entryway to health and wellness. The locations of these points closely correspond to the body points associated with the motor cortex and the chakras that are scanned during the rotation of consciousness during yoga nidra. This involvement of the marma points adds another healing dimension to the practice.

## Guided Imagery for the Mental/Emotional Stage (Mano Maya Kosha)

Guided imagery, sometimes referred to as creative visualization, is like intentional daydreaming. The difference is that in daydreaming the mind is allowed to go wherever it pleases. Instead of this, the mind is gently directed in a specific and special manner. This mindbody technique is found in yoga and is called *bhavana*; it works well with yoga nidra. Guided imagery can be used for relaxation, healing, magnifying the positive aspects of the mindbody connection, and evoking intuition. During our experience, guided imagery is used for balancing and enhancing the health of the chakras and for sparking intuition.

Guided imagery does not necessarily mean "mentally seeing pictures." Rather, any of the senses can be used during a guided imagery exercise. For example, a guided imagery exercise might ask you to focus on a setting or environment that feels safe and comfortable. This can be experienced and accomplished by mentally seeing the setting, or getting a concept or impression of it, feeling or sensing the environment, or using the senses of sound or smell. As Belleruth Naparstek, the author of *Staying Well with Guided Imagery*, says, "There are many right ways to experience guided imagery." Therefore, use whatever naturally works for you.

The principle and practice of cultivating the positive, or *pratipaksha bhavana*, is used in the guided imagery exercise in this chapter. It comes from Yoga Sutra II.33 and advises us to cultivate the positive when we are troubled by negative thoughts and feelings. See appendix 3 for more information about cultivating the positive and a meditation dedicated to it.

## Guided Imagery for the Intuitive Stage
## (Vijnana Maya Kosha)

Guided imagery is used for enhancing the conditions for intuitive wisdom and for inner knowing to be facilitated. This provides the opportunity for receiving direct, intelligent guidance with respect to something that would be helpful for you to know about yourself, gain an understanding about a situation, or reveal an answer to something that may be causing confusion. This provides a wonderful opportunity for the wisdom you may have been searching for to reveal itself.

## Guided Imagery for Feeling Peace and Joy
## (Ananda Maya Kosha)

Guided imagery can also be used as a stepping-off point into experiencing a profound sense of unconditional peace and joy. This can naturally guide us into the timeless, spacious, and blissful experience of the *Atma*.

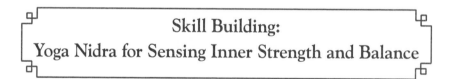

# Skill Building:
# Yoga Nidra for Sensing Inner Strength and Balance

The audio version of this exercise is available for download so that you can experience the full benefits without having to read the script. Eventually, you will be able to guide yourself from memory. Reminders are given in chapter 3 for getting the most out of your yoga nidra experience. Follow the tips in appendix 4 if you are leading others.

# Part 1: Readiness and Reminders

Choose a quiet place. One where you'll feel comfortable and are unlikely to be disturbed.

Get your props ready, shut the door, dim the lights, and turn off the phone or whatever else might be distracting.

## Relaxation Pose (Shavasana)

Let's get ready to experience yoga nidra. Lie down on your back, aligning your head, neck, and spine. If you like, use a thin cushion under your head and a cover for your comfort. Move your shoulders down from your ears and tuck your shoulder blades in comfortably. Place your arms out to your sides with your palms up. Have your legs uncrossed and out straight. Make sure the insides of your legs don't touch. If you prefer, put your feet flat on the floor with your knees up.

Please close your eyes or have them slightly open. Mentally, let yourself know that it's time to experience the rest, relaxation, and renewal of yoga nidra... Make yourself as comfortable as possible.

In your own way, remind yourself of the value of relaxation and to stay awake... Let your experience be natural and effortless. Needless distractions will be easy to handle. Feel free to add your own reminders now.

# Part 2: Setting a Sankalpa

This is the time for making your sankalpa. It's a consistent statement that can express a positive quality that's personally beneficial, or affirm a change in your behavior for the better, or reflect something meaningful you'd like to do with your one, precious life. Something to ignite your energy so your spirit soars.

If you wish, use this time to formulate your resolve now. Keep it clear, brief, and sincere. Be consistent by using the same one from one practice to the next. Silently say yours in a heartfelt way a few times... Imagine what it'd be like if this was already happening.

[Pause]

Take a big breath in and let it go.

Remind yourself to stay aware and alert. If you'd like to make any adjustments for more comfort, feel free to do it now.

[Pause]

## Part 3: Yoga Nidra in Six Stages

### Stage 1: Body Scanning and Rotation of Consciousness for Physical Relaxation (Anna Maya Kosha)

**Sensory Awareness**

Notice where the back of your head touches the surface supporting it, having a direct experience of the contact point where your head meets the surface...letting the surface completely support your head.

It's time to open your mouth a little and gently move your jaw up and down and around. Easy does it... Now, let your mouth rest and close your lips, allowing your teeth to part slightly and the corners of your lips to soften and relax. There's no need for any facial expression, so let any muscular tightness or holding fade away.

Let's be more attentive to your senses, bringing them alive. Please focus your attention on your eyes. Keeping them closed, lift and lower your eyebrows a few times... Now, let yourself become still.

Become aware of your eyes resting in their sockets... Sense the outside air on your eyelids...and become aware of how your eyelids touch and cover your eyeballs, like eyeshades. Even though your eyes are closed, you can still see. Start focusing your inner vision and watch whatever appears on the inside shade of your eyelids, coming and going. It might appear dark, there may be some color, perhaps some shapes... It doesn't really matter what's there—what matters is watching whatever comes and goes... There's no need for making comments about it... Let your eyes rest now and become still, yet watching the inner space...simply looking and softly gazing and watching in stillness.

[Pause]

To enhance hearing awareness, begin noticing the sounds you're now hearing... Start focusing on the distant sounds...simply taking in these sounds... There's no need to name them, or even to prefer one sound over another...letting the sounds come to you.

[Pause, thirty to sixty seconds]

And now, listening to the nearby sounds right around you...letting them come and go...listening effortlessly to the nearby sounds... And now, listening to the sound of your own breathing...noticing the air coming and going...and how it sounds... You might be aware of other internal sounds...simply listening with curiosity, openness, and acceptance, listening without reacting or naming the sounds...

And expanding your awareness from the sounds of breathing...and blending the nearby and faraway sounds, like listening peripherally, letting them all blend together...and into the background... And continue listening to the instructions being given. Staying alert and aware yet relaxing and feeling calmer and calmer.

## Rotation of Consciousness

It's time to mentally pay a visit to various areas of the body... It's fine to silently repeat each location to yourself as you mentally follow along. There's no need for any movements as you follow along.

It's time to mentally find your right hand...sensing where your right hand is, finding your right hand mentally...your entire right hand...and the right thumb...the pointer finger...the middle finger...the ring finger...and the baby finger...the palm of the hand...the back of the hand...the wrist...the lower arm...elbow... upper arm...right shoulder...the armpit...down the right side to the hip...upper leg...knee...calf muscle...ankle...heel...bottom of the foot...top of the foot...the big toe...the second toe...the third toe...the fourth toe...and the baby toe...and now the whole entire foot...the whole entire foot.

And now, mentally find your left hand...sensing your left hand, finding your left hand mentally...your entire left hand...the left thumb...the pointer finger...the middle finger...the ring finger... and the baby finger...the palm of the hand...the back of the hand... the wrist...the lower arm...elbow...upper arm...left shoulder...the armpit...down the left side to the hip...upper leg...knee...calf muscle...ankle...heel...bottom of the foot...top of the foot...the big toe...the second toe...the third toe...the fourth toe...and the baby toe...and now the whole entire foot...the whole entire foot... having a direct experience of your whole foot.

If you get distracted, simply bring your attention back to what we're doing. Remember to stay alert and aware.

Moving your awareness now to the base of your spine...up to your lower back...midback...and upper back...to the top of your head... and now to the center of the forehead...

[Pause fifteen seconds]

And now to the right eyebrow...left eyebrow...right eyeball...left eyeball...right eye socket...left eye socket...right eyelid...left eyelid...and the line between your eyelids... letting your eyes rest... And now the right ear...the left ear...right cheek...left cheek...the nose...and the tip of the nose...the upper lip...the lower lip...the line between the lips...and the corners of the lips... And now the jaw...and going inside the mouth...sensing the inside of the mouth...the tongue...gums...teeth...feeling the moisture, actually feeling the moisture...and tasting the taste, just tasting the taste... and now to the throat...the heart...the upper abdomen...the navel...the lower abdomen...and the base of the spine.

Can you notice yourself sensing a feeling of calmness coupled with alertness?

[Pause thirty seconds]

Remember to stay aware and remain alert.

And now to the right leg, the whole and entire right leg...all the parts of the whole right leg, all at once... And now to the left leg, the whole and entire left leg...and all the parts of the whole left leg, all at once... And sensing both legs at the same time...sensing both legs.

And now to the right arm, the whole and entire right arm...all the parts of the whole right arm at once... And now to the left arm, the whole and entire left arm...and all the parts of the whole left arm at once... And both arms at the same time...sensing both arms...both hands...and both arms and hands.

And moving on to sensing your head...and now your face...and both the head and face at the same time...the head and face together.

And now having a direct experience of the back side of your body...sensing the contact points where the back side of your body touches the surface it's on...picking them all out...feeling them... and now, experiencing the whole back side of your body at once... And now the front side of your body...the whole and entire front side of your body...perhaps feeling the textures of your clothes touching your skin...and sensing the air touching your skin...and both the front and back side of your body all at once...and all together at the same time.

This is the time to sense your whole self, your whole body all at once...all together now...sensing your whole body at the same time... Notice if it feels heavy and still, being totally relaxed, yet fully awake... Perhaps, sensing the space around your body...and now the body and the space around it simultaneously.

If you would like to shift around or make adjustments, do so.

## Stage 2: Breathing and Chakra Meditation (Prana Maya Kosha)

### Breathing Meditation

Now, we go to the breath...move your awareness to the ongoing and natural breath; there's no need to change it...just feeling the breath as it comes and goes...again and again, remaining aware of breathing and little else...and letting any mental chatter dissolve into the background, focusing mostly on your breathing...following the soothing breath, over and over...noticing how soft and subtle it is.

Now it's time to notice where it's easiest to monitor your breath...it could be how it sounds, or how it feels at your nostrils...perhaps in your throat...or the upper, middle, or lower part of your lungs... simply noticing wherever your breath is most prominent...it really doesn't matter where, just let your attention and awareness rest wherever your breath is most noticeable now…and if distractions come…simply bring your attention back to the breath…anchoring your attention on breathing.

[Pause]

And now, please rest your attention at the forehead…let your attention remain at the brow.

[Pause]

## Chakra Meditation

And now, you can start using your mind's eye, if you wish, for remembering and imagining a few scenarios. Use whatever senses make this easy for you. Some people can visualize and "see" things, many don't. It might be easier to conceptualize, or feel, or use the sense of smell or taste. Sometimes, the scenarios will change on their own in order to match your needs more closely; if so, just let it happen. And if you're not in the mood for this, or scenarios are illusive, or something entirely different comes up, that's fine too. If you prefer, feel free to linger on a scenario or two—or change it on your own, picking back up whenever you like. Go with this in the spirit of curiosity, accepting and trusting what's happening for you, and with the heart of a neutral, yet compassionate observer.

Let your attention start running up and down the entire spine from the top of the head to the base of the spine…circling up and down…up and down…connecting with the energetic power centers within…connecting with the chakras.

## Root Chakra

Become aware of a time, place, or circumstance for feeling completely comfortable, safe, and protected. It can come from a memory, or from using your imagination to make something up; or maybe you're feeling it right now. Bring it alive in your mind's eye, sensing it now, a feeling of being completely comfortable and protected... How does it look?...What does it feel like?... Were there sounds or smells involved? Sensing what it's like to feel secure and protected. Embellish it any way you want so that you're feeling more and more secure and protected... And noticing how and where feeling secure and protected feels in your body. Welcoming in whatever you experience.

## Sacral Chakra

Now, draw your awareness to a time, circumstance, or place of experiencing your senses, engrossed in what you were seeing, feeling, smelling, or tasting. Perhaps it was out in nature, like watching the sky. Or maybe you were doing something with someone, or experiencing something special. Make it a time when you felt fully present and aware of what you were feeling and sensing. Feeling emotionally alive, sensual...creative... And noticing whatever your experience is right now. Noticing how it shows up mentally and physically.

## Solar Plexus Chakra

Bring to mind a situation when you felt really good about yourself... when you felt on top of the world...happy about an accomplishment, possibly feeling really confident. Use your mind's eye to bring it back alive... And noticing how it feels in your body now, sensing it, here and now, physically, mentally, and emotionally. Welcoming into awareness whatever you experience.

## Heart Chakra

This time, recall being loving, compassionate. It could be loving or compassionate toward a person, a pet, or something else. Any affectionate feeling, a fondness. What's important is feeling loving...and experiencing it again now... And how about a time when you felt really loved...so cared for and lovable, a time when you felt loved, supported, and accepted, just for who you are... Use your imagination to feel it now and sensing how this impacts your body and mind. And noticing how this feels, noticing what you're feeling right now. Welcoming in whatever you're experiencing. Staying with whatever you're experiencing.

**Throat Chakra**

Now it's time to become aware of being completely understood... If you like, use your mind's eye to sense being able to easily communicate clearly, kindly, and honestly...and able to understand what's being communicated with you, deeply listening, understanding... And noticing what you're feeling right now.

[Pause]

## Stage 3: Relaxing Mentally and Emotionally
## (Mano Maya Kosha)

It's time for reflecting on your experience of these scenarios. Trusting in what happened, or what may not have happened... trusting whatever was encountered and revealed. Taking in the sweetness, the surprises, and the paradoxes...and letting areas that may be calling out for further exploration to rise to the surface. Welcoming the images, the thoughts, the feelings, and all the rest. And knowing that it's not even necessary to have to fix or solve anything but to simply hold awareness in a gentle, accepting kind of way, relaxing into it, more and more... Reflecting.

[Pause]

## Stage 4: Experiencing Intuition (Vijnana Maya Kosha)

### Third-Eye Chakra

And now, continuing to be at ease and resting in awareness, it's time for welcoming in fresh perspectives, insights, and new understandings...and being ready to receive intuitive guidance that can come now or perhaps later. Being open and receptive now...and having insights about something that's helpful for you.

[Pause]

## Stage 5: Experiencing Joyfulness (Ananda Maya Kosha)

Being in the present, notice whatever you're experiencing. Perhaps it's a sense of inner peace, of delight, of deep satisfaction. If it's helpful, use your mind's eye to experience feelings of pleasure, a time of contentment, of happiness... Perhaps a time when you laughed so hard you could barely stop...or the feeling of jumping for joy...bringing the feelings back alive...and noticing how these sensations and feelings can be relived now... And, if you like, let the memory fade away...not having to rely on events, things, or anything else for being aware of sensations of contentment, joyfulness, and ease, and being in touch with this constant inner joy that is always and already yours.

[Pause]

## Stage 6: Atma Awareness

### Crown Chakra

And now expanding your awareness and settling into a feeling of being connected, of belonging, perhaps sensing deep contentment... Oneness and wholeness. Resting in pure, limitless awareness.

[Long, silent pause]

## Part 4: Remembering Your Sankalpa

Om shanti—peace, peace, peace... Now it's time to remember your sankalpa. Repeat the same sankalpa made at the beginning. Say it with your heart several times... Imagine how it would be if it were already so.

[Pause]

Take a full breath in...and let it go.

## Part 5: Transition Back to Full Awareness

And now become more and more aware of your whole self... What're you experiencing?... And sensing that now. What're you noticing?...Perhaps it's feeling completely peaceful and quiet, yet so refreshed and full of delight. Welcoming what's happening now.

And notice your soft and subtle breathing...in and out...in and out.

Becoming more and more aware of the whole body, lying here and experiencing peaceful, relaxing, and joyful energy.

[Pause]

It's time to come back into full awareness and wakefulness, and to bring back with you all the benefits of yoga nidra to help yourself as well as to benefit others. Becoming more and more aware of this time and place...sensing this moment in time and these surroundings. You're becoming very clear-headed and so wide awake, and noticing how you're feeling totally relaxed and refreshed.

Become increasingly more aware of your presence in these surroundings: what's above...what's all around...and sensing what's below... When you're ready, begin moving your body, stretching it however you wish to... It's time to get ready to roll over onto your side... Okay now, roll over and curl up into a comfortable position.

[Pause]

It's time to use your arms to bring yourself into a comfortable and upright sitting position... Touch the tips of your thumbs to the tips of your index fingers and rest your hands on your knees. Soak it in.

[Pause]

Blink your eyes open. Inhale deeply and let it go... Notice if you're smiling.

Remember, the best results come with regular practice. You'll be blessed with better health, a clear and balanced mind, emotional stability, kindness, and more. Keep your sankalpa in mind and allow it to take root and flourish in your daily life.

## Variations

**Use different hand positions (mudras).** Supplement your experience by using some of the mudras outlined in appendix 1. Add the *kubera mudra* when setting your sankalpa. The *hakini mudra* can be used during the breath awareness stage, as it helps balance the chakras.

**Lengthen the sensory or body scans.** Spend extra time exploring more details as you go along. For instance, you could spend more time within the mouth by noticing the roof of the mouth, the floor of the mouth, the inside cheeks, different aspects of the tongue, the gums and teeth, how it tastes, the moisture, and so on. Get into it.

**Shorten the sensory or body scans.** Either omit some of the details or combine various areas. For instance, instead of dwelling on the component parts, become aware of your whole hand at once rather than going through each finger, and so on. Just remember that your goal is to experience yoga nidra rather than looking for ways to rush through it. If it works, keep it up.

**Use affirmations and mantras.** Mentally say an affirmation or repeat a mantra at each area during the body scan or in conjunction with your breath. Options include silently repeating your sankalpa; mentally saying, "Health and happiness"; or repeating "Om" or "Peaceful and calm." The ones that follow are based on the chakras. Say them silently to yourself, using some or all of them depending on your needs and the time available. While each phrase appears only once, be sure to take enough time to connect with each one, particularly the ones that hold the most meaning for you. Feel free to modify the wording until you find the version that feels right. Keep it positive and in the present tense.

> *Root chakra:* "I am secure, steady, and strong. I am centered."

> *Sacral chakra:* "I experience my feelings and emotions, and express intimacy. I am sensual and creative."

> *Solar plexus chakra:* "I am happy and healthy in body, mind, and soul. I am confident."

> *Heart chakra:* "My heart flows with compassion for myself and others. I am lovable and loving."

> *Throat chakra:* "I communicate clearly, kindly, and listen deeply. I am self-expressive."

> *Third-eye chakra:* "I trust my instincts and insights. I am intuitive."

> *Crown chakra:* "I am connected with the sacred. I am."

**Use a different breathing meditation.** If you prefer, the breathing meditations from chapters 4 or 6 could be substituted. Others are found in appendix 2.

**Vary the guided imagery exercise to suit your needs.** Instead of practicing them all at once as written during the stage 2, take your time with the one that holds special meaning to you. Feel free to stay with it for as long as you want and practice it as often as you like. Save the others for later.

**Use guided imagery exercises for healing.** Use imagery scenarios that center on healing in the second stage of part 3. Here are some examples:

- Remember a time when you felt full of health and energy. Take time to relive that experience by remembering what you were doing (hiking, gardening, singing, enjoying others, dancing, playing sports, and so on). Bring it alive by using as many of your senses as you can by reliving what it was like—but in the present time. Finally, imagine feeling full of health and energy in the future.

- Use your imagination to sense yourself healing. For example, if your shoulder is sore from stress, imagine the soreness fading away by using your breathing; center your attention on your shoulder and feel the stress and the soreness being taken away each time you exhale. Give yourself enough time to feel it being effective. Next, you could imagine healing energy restoring it. Finish by imagining yourself using your shoulder freely and easily.

**Release mental, emotional, and limiting beliefs.** Substitute the pairing of opposites exercise in part 3, stage 3, in chapter 6 in place of the guided imagery.

# What to Remember

- The mindbody connection has the capacity to heal stress when given the right conditions, namely deep rest and relaxation as is experienced with yoga nidra during the rotation of consciousness and breath awareness.

- The map of consciousness, wisely based on the sensory-motor cortex and the chakras, is used for the body scan. It is extremely relaxing and healing while it boosts awareness.

- All of us have seven primary energy centers called chakras that span from the base of the spine to the top of the head. They guide the well-being of our body, mind, emotions, and spirit. Yoga nidra provides us with a method to balance our chakras, reduce stress, and make positive changes.

- Guided imagery is like intentional daydreaming, but it uses the power of the mind for stress relief, relaxation, healing, behavior change, and sparking intuition. Guided imagery can be experienced in many ways. Some people can visualize and see images. Having an inner sense, impression, or mental concept comes easier to others. Feeling, hearing, and tasting are other ways guided imagery can be experienced. Use whatever comes easiest for you, whether it uses a combination or a single method.

- None of this works unless you practice. Regularity matters.

- Lean toward inner strength.

## Chapter 6

# Revitalization: Yoga Nidra for High-Level Living

As your yoga nidra practice advances, it becomes possible to develop much more control over the autonomic nervous system and a range of reactions to stress. This next experience enables us to be less reactionary to stress and to respond with more ease and equanimity when stressful events occur. Emotional and mental issues are eased away, and clarity of mind shines through to reveal one's inner core of peaceful steadiness. Recovery from the onslaught of stress happens much faster as well. A healthier perspective is developed and can be put to use. For instance, one's *sankalpa* (resolve) and other inner resources are readily available to help lessen the impact of stress and the identification with it.

As Paul, a student of yoga nidra, puts it, "My fuse is longer, and the things that used to bug me rarely do anymore. For once, I am noticing the beauty around me, like sunsets, instead of being caught up and stressed out. I'm enjoying life much more."

This next yoga nidra experience will use techniques based on moment-to-moment awareness training, autogenic training, the paradox of opposites, and the awareness of witnessing one's experience. Let's explore each of these techniques and why they work before practicing them.

# Moment-to-Moment Awareness and the Steadiness of Mind

The sixth limb of Raja (Ashtanga) yoga is *dharana* and refers to concentration and steadiness of mind. Meditation, or *dhyana*, is the seventh limb. (Refer to chapter 2 for a review of the concept.) Concentration, mindfulness, and awareness training are meditative techniques and states of awareness—and are all slightly different facets of the same gem. Each has its roots in the moment-to-moment awareness of the here and now. Each facet has its place in stress prevention and treatment. Each holds a promise and a pathway to uncovering the heart of one's true Self and revealing inner peace, steadiness, self-understanding, and joyful living. We will refer to the benefits of these meditative techniques as the *awareness advantage*. Receptivity, acceptance, and the impartial awareness of witness consciousness with the capacity to tap in to one's inner smarts are developed.

## The Awareness Advantage

Making some time to choose a focal point, practice awareness training, hone concentration skills, and benefit from relaxation training through yoga nidra is well worth it. These skills benefit you by turning the relaxation response on while turning the harmful effects of the stress reaction off. The awareness advantage begins seeping into your day.

Let's look at this from the standpoint of the *koshas*, the layers covering our true Self. Muscular tightness in the neck and shoulders is now noticed and released before it becomes a headache (*anna maya kosha*). Instead of blowing it, it gets easier to calm down and reclaim energy by breathing more deeply (*prana maya kosha*). The awareness advantage of paying attention on a moment-to-moment basis improves memory, calms mental and emotional turmoil, and reduces limiting beliefs (*mano maya kosha*). For instance, increased mental awareness lowers the odds of losing things, which can range from items around the house to your mental or emotional health. The constant and useless struggle that comes from trying to hold on to the good and avoid the bad is better controlled. Daily dramas, real or imagined, happen less frequently and are more easily dealt with when they are seen for what they are and handled from a better perspective. Intuition comes to the forefront to assist with finding answers that are based on truth (*vijnana maya kosha*). More energy is available for enjoying life (*ananda maya kosha*). Inner peace and Self-understanding become pervasive (*Atma*).

Sandy, a working mother of three, said, "Yoga nidra is where I find myself turning when I need solace or need to resolve an issue. There's a clarity that comes with the practice and a feeling of being enveloped by spirit."

## Increasing Concentration, Awareness, Emotional Balance, and Peace of Mind

The awareness advantage improves through practicing yoga nidra. The mindbody is retrained for alertness, composure, and high-level living. Don't let the explanation of the following components be daunting. It is given to help you understand how and why this works so well. All that is really needed is to go through the yoga nidra exercise and experience it for yourself. Remember the yoga sutras' emphasis on practice and non-attachment to results. Just do it, drop your judgments, let go of expectations, and be more observant in an impartial manner.

### Autogenic Training

Autogenic training, developed by Johannes Schultz and Wolfgang Luthe in the 1930s, is another effective technique to lower stress and reduce anxiety. This technique is still widely used and respected today. It has the capacity to increase body awareness and bring automatic, unconscious physical reactions under control. Since the autogenic training technique has such a powerful and positive affect on the parasympathetic nervous system, it effectively turns the stress reaction off and the relaxation response on. In a meta-analysis of clinical outcome studies on autogenic training, it was shown to help treat tension head-aches and migraines, mild to moderate hypertension (high blood pressure), coronary heart disease, asthma, pain management, anxiety disorders, mild to moderate depression or dysthymia, and functional sleep disorders. Autogenic training has positive effects on mood, cognitive performance, and quality of life (Stetter and Kupper 2002). In addition, autogenic training teaches your body to respond to helpful verbal commands and demonstrates the temporary nature of sensations. This process is physiological and not magical or mystical.

To do it, statements are repeated silently until the desired effect occurs. Traditionally, these statements first center on producing the physical sensations of heaviness and feelings of warmth in the arms and legs. The feeling of heaviness generates muscular relaxation as your body responds to these suggestions. As the sensation of heaviness in the body becomes habituated, the sensation of physical lightness occurs spontaneously, since the brain is no longer interested in the physical body and is freed of it. Typically, more statements are then used to calm and steady the heartbeat and breath, soften and warm the stomach, and cool the forehead. It is quite empowering to be able to create these physical reactions in the body that are normally unconscious and automatic. All in all, the awareness advantage increases.

This next yoga nidra process uses autogenic training to take advantage of *habituation* and build upon it by using the technique to experience opposite sensations for balancing feelings, emotions, and beliefs, and then to couple it with the practice of witnessing the experience.

## Habituation

Habituation is a physiological and emotional process during which a stimulus no longer causes a response. It is a type of learning that goes on in animals and humans and occurs naturally and unconsciously. It helps us ignore neutral stimuli that neither help nor hurt us by filtering out what's irrelevant. This way, more important things can be dealt with. Distractions move to the background and out of awareness. In other words, habituation occurs whenever you get used to something that had been new or foreign at first. Here are a couple of examples:

- Certain noises are nerve-racking at first: a loud lawn mower, busy traffic, honking horns. But these same noises seem to fade away after a while, even though they are still happening at the same frequency and volume. In other words, it is like when you notice the quiet after the dishwasher or air conditioner shuts off.

- When stepping into a room for the first time, the primary thing you might notice is a strong smell: antiseptic cleanser, a burning candle, something baking. Even when those things continue to give off an aroma, their smell goes unnoticed after a while.

Let's do a quick experiment on habituation. Clasp your hands together and interlace your fingers. Hold this for a few seconds. Next, interlace your fingers the other way: If your left thumb was on top, put the right one on top and move all the fingers over by one down the line. Notice how this feels to you. Does it feel weird? If you held your hands like this for a little bit habituation would happen, and having your hands this way would start feeling normal again. Before too long, it would go unnoticed.

So what does this have to do with stress relief and yoga nidra? Someone who is under constant stress "forgets" that he or she is tense due to habituation and no longer notices it consciously, even though everyone else might see it plain as day. The tension may only become noticeable after it causes physical problems like muscular tension, insomnia, or hypertension—or when emotional and behavioral problems arise, like losing one's temper. Sometimes the tension becomes noticeable once it is gone, like when the pressure lifts when on vacation.

Practicing feeling heaviness and the resulting relaxation during autogenic training, for example, becomes habituated, and the heavy feelings start going unnoticed and start feeling light instead. The awareness advantage increases—and the longer the exposure, the faster this occurs. Habituation is helpful since energy is no longer wasted when something is not really causing a problem but is still available if danger does arise.

When Chris, a college student, recently moved into a new neighborhood, everything seemed strange to him at first. For starters, the neighbor's barking dog kept him up at night. After a while, he got used to it and he could sleep through the noise. Eventually, the dog got used to having Chris next door and quit barking unnecessarily.

Habituation is constantly taking place and happens without our being aware of it. The next yoga nidra experience takes it out of the unconscious realm and makes it conscious. The principle of habituation is put to work through the exposure to and the experience of different physical sensations, emotions, and beliefs. Your ability to concentrate will increase.

Most of the time, the majority of us try to ignore or avoid whatever is disturbing or stressful. But if we really allow ourselves to feel muscular tension consciously, tense muscles will no longer be troublesome, as tension is resolved when it arises and is noticed instead of ignored. This happens during meditation too. Having a tired back from sitting erect gets distracting. Rather than immediately moving or giving up, the sore muscles will often go away on their own when they are given proper attention until the distraction solves itself. In the next exercise, the mindbody settles down when the brain gets bored with (habituated to) paying nonjudgmental attention to sounds as they come and go. The peacefulness of awareness without words results.

If you would like to try this right now, find a place that feels tense and use habituation on purpose to notice what happens. For instance, if you are aware of tension in your jaw, without changing it focus on it by noticing how it actually feels when clenching your teeth; feel the muscular tension in your cheeks, lips, chin, or tongue. Most likely, it will release, melting away on its own. If it doesn't, take the necessary action needed for relief. Either way, tension and stress are released.

## The Paradox of Opposites

A *paradox* incorporates the concept of both/and. Take the night sky, for example. There is the sky and the moon, but for the night sky to exist, *both* the sky *and* the moon are needed. In other words, both the combined parts and the individual parts are needed. This sentence is composed of separate words, but all the words are needed to express something.

Likewise, a paradox is something that seems real on the surface but really isn't. Our stressful feelings, thoughts, and emotions certainly seem real when they are happening but are actually temporary. We mistake what is changeable (koshas) for what is real (Atma), even though what is changeable exists. The koshas and the Atma have a both/and relationship.

The idea of *opposites* incorporates two different, contrary, and separate sides or positions. For there to be an awareness of darkness, there must be awareness of light. To recognize peace, one must know stress. For there to be right, there must be wrong. The same goes for heaviness/lightness, noise/quiet, joy/sorrow, and pain/pleasure. The *paradox of opposites* comes into play with the awareness and pairing of opposite physical sensations, emotions, and beliefs to aid healing, become beneficial through habituation, and advance the awareness advantage.

To understand one thing, its opposite must also be understood. It seems wrong to delve into stress, but it is the right thing to do under the right circumstances. Stress, when truly explored in the context and safety of witness consciousness and a calm mind, will eventually become habituated and dissolve into peace and calmness. Three things may happen during this process. First, it may disappear temporarily or more completely. Second, it may stay the same temporarily, providing a strong focus to rest and develop stable witness consciousness. Third, it may increase temporarily, serving as a sign that what is being contacted is purifying and releasing at the root. On the other hand, if we try to hold on to peace due to the fear of losing it, stress will enter the picture. Soon, we will briefly touch on the principle of karma as well as Newton's third law of physics that says, "For every action, there is an equal and opposite reaction." The next experience will put all this to the test so you can prove or disprove these concepts for yourself.

The parts of the brain responsible for maintaining harmony between the opposites of inner and outer world awareness are stimulated during a stage of yoga nidra as various physical sensations—like heaviness/lightness, coolness/warmth, stress/calmness—are made conscious. Homeostatic balance, according to the book *Yoga Nidra* (Saraswati 1998, 39), is maintained and even evolves by bringing normally involuntary and unconscious functions under control and establishing new neuronal circuitry, so contradictory states of emotional awareness are maintained in a relaxed state of witness awareness. In this way, yoga nidra progressively transforms our total experience of sensory life with repeated practice.

The book goes on to say that the pairing of opposite physical sensations, emotions, and so on harmonizes the opposite hemispheres of the brain and helps in balancing our basic drives. Emotional relaxation naturally occurs as memories of profound feelings are relived and alleviated through habituation. This practice also deepens receptivity and willpower. Limiting and outdated beliefs are corrected.

Newton's third law of physics comes into play here. If it is true that "For every action, there is an equal and opposite reaction," both sides of every pair of opposites are bound to come up. Karma, the yogic principle of cause and effect, suggests that we create our own reality (stress/ peace, action/reaction) depending on the choices we make in how we perceive and respond in the world and because thought, word, and deed are linked: For example, an endless loop of happy/sad/happy/sad/ happy/sad goes on and on. This points to the temporary nature and the continuous cycle of opposing feelings, thoughts, and emotions. Plus, experiencing either one or the other half of the pair keeps us lopsided and trapped in the cycle.

During yoga nidra, we are guided to step back from the immediate experience of the pairs to gain a new and expanded perspective by welcoming each half one at a time. Healing and integration occurs when both halves of the pair are experienced from a welcoming perspective rather than one of resisting or clinging to one or the other. Gradually, each part of the pair is experienced simultaneously and with witness consciousness. Experiencing all this also reminds us that we can choose what we want to pay attention to and from what perspective. Practicing this equanimity during yoga nidra eventually transfers itself into daily life so that acceptance of the wide range of life experiences is encountered more peacefully and with greater awareness and ease.

This starts working when we consciously experience a specific physical sensation, feeling, or belief until we become habituated. This causes its opposite to naturally and spontaneously appear until habituation happens again. Eventually the thinking mind becomes bored and both pairs are felt simultaneously. Neutrally witnessing the experience is also practiced along the way. This eventually reveals the inner dimension (Atma) that is changeless and always present. As progressive parts of the exercise are practiced, we help this expanded awareness and perspective along by consciously spending time shifting back and forth between the opposites with stepping back and being Present to all that is happening. In this way, the temporary nature of sensory experience is realized and understood, the opposites merge into oneness, the sense of separation dissolves into wholeness, and unwavering peace is experienced (Atma).

## Putting these Principles into Practice

Stress is deeply relieved the more you directly experience the temporary nature of thoughts, beliefs, and feelings, as well as the permanent nature, wholeness, and Presence of the Atma.

To experiment with and explore the nature of habituation, try this: the next time a noise, for example, is getting the best of you, use awareness training to impartially listen to it as sound; take a stance of neutral curiosity toward it and let the annoyance drop away as the noise fades from conscious awareness. Another option is to become curious and fully aware of feeling annoyed, including the physical sensations and the mental chatter taking place. Instead of identifying personally with the feelings, practice curiosity. Watch your stress levels decrease.

Personalize this next practice by going back to the Assess Your Stress survey in chapter 1. Get your journal out and divide the page into two columns. In the first column, write down the physical sensations, feelings, beliefs, and emotional items you checked off. In the next column, write down the opposite qualities that counter what is listed. Finally, choose a pair that you want to work with during this yoga nidra experience.

## Skill Building:
## Yoga Nidra For High-Level Living

Be sure to download the audio recording so you can reap the full benefits of the following practice. If needed, review the reminders given in chapter 3 for getting the most out of your yoga nidra experience. Tips for leading others are in appendix 4.

## Part 1: Readiness and Reminders

Choose a comfortable place where you're unlikely to be disturbed. Get your props ready, close the door, lower the lights, turn off the phone, and limit anything else to minimize distractions. This introduction and the instructions on *shavasana* can be omitted once you're familiar with both.

### Relaxation Pose (Shavasana)

Lie down on a blanket or mat on a firm surface. Use a thin cushion under your head, and cover up with a blanket if desired. Enjoy stretching if you like.

Close your eyes whenever you're ready. Maximize your comfort by positioning your head so that your chin is slightly tucked down. Line up your head, neck, and spine. Adjust your hair if it's in the way. Move your shoulders down from your ears and position your shoulder blades underneath for comfort and support. Stretch out your arms so they aren't touching the sides of your body, with your palms facing up. Notice your low back and hips. Adjust their position so there's enough room under there, and so it feels even and balanced. Straighten your legs out. To help ease tensions in the back, hips, and legs, have your heels stretched apart so that the inside of your legs don't touch. Otherwise, use a firm pillow under your legs. Let your feet rest. Give yourself a few moments to settle in… Take a big breath in and sigh it out… This is your time to relax and let go. Make any further adjustments to your clothes, props, and position for maximum comfort and minimum distractions. Give yourself some personal reminders to enhance your experience.

## Part 2: Setting a Sankalpa

Let's begin. It's time to set your sankalpa. It's something from deep inside that sparks your energy and warms your heart. It's used to improve a behavior, develop a positive quality, support spirituality, or reflect something you'd like that gives meaning and purpose to your life direction. If you don't have one, let this be the moment to let one come to you, otherwise start recalling yours now. Be consistent and use the one that you've established, giving it time to take root, grow, and thrive. Keep it brief and say it in the present tense as if it's already happened. Silently repeat yours about three times with heartfelt conviction… Sense what it'd be like if it were already happening.

[Pause]

Take a big breath in, and sigh it out.

# Part 3: Yoga Nidra in Six Stages

## *Stage 1: Autogenic Training for Physical Relaxation (Anna Maya Kosha)*

Feel free to adjust your position for more comfort and ease… Bring your attention to your mouth. Start moving your jaw all around to release tension—let it go up and down, side to side, and all around. Let your mouth rest with your teeth parted slightly. Moisten your lips if you wish, and allow the corners of your lips to soften more and more.

Take a nice big breath in through your nose, and sigh it out through your mouth. Do this a few more times at your own pace.

[Pause]

Become more aware of the surrounding sounds…listening and blending the sounds, letting them come to you from far and near, being as receptive as you can rather than preferring one or another… And continue listening to the instructions being offered.

Even though your eyes are closed, squeeze and release your eyelids a few times…and let them rest.

Take your attention to your right arm. Repeat these phrases silently after me: *My right arm is getting heavy… My right arm is getting heavier and heavier… My right arm is very heavy…* and let it happen, feeling the heaviness in your arm…*My right arm is very, very heavy. It's relaxing more and more.*

Bring your attention to your right leg. Please silently repeat after me: *My right leg is getting heavy… My right leg is getting heavier and heavier… My right leg is very heavy…* and let it happen, feeling the heaviness in your right leg…*My right leg is very, very heavy…and relaxing more and more, heavier and heavier.*

If distractions arise, bring your attention back again and again.

Take your attention to your left arm. Repeating and responding: *My left arm is getting heavy... My left arm is getting heavier and heavier... My left arm is very heavy...*and let it happen, feeling the heaviness in your arm... *My left arm is very, very heavy. It's relaxing more and more.*

Bring your attention to your left leg. Please silently repeat after me: *My left leg is getting heavy... My left leg is getting heavier and heavier... My left leg is very heavy...*and let it happen, feeling the heaviness in your left leg... *My left leg is very, very heavy...and relaxing more and more.*

*My whole body is getting heavier and heavier... My body is very heavy... My body is very, very heavy...and relaxing more and more.* And let it happen, feeling the sensations in your whole body. There's no need to try and make anything happen. Perhaps noticing the earth's magnetic pull, and sinking fully into it... And if at any time you notice that your body starts feeling light and buoyant, let it happen. Simply noticing and allowing your experience.

Remind yourself in your own way to remain alert, awake, and Present.

## Stage 2: Relax Energetically (Prana Maya Kosha)

Now, it's time to bring awareness to your breathing. Leave it alone and let it be just as it is, as you follow the passage of the air coming and going through your nose... Allow your breathing to be effortless. Each time your mind wanders, just bring it back to breathing.

Just for now, start noticing how the air feels cool inside your nostrils when it's going in...simply noticing the coolness each time the air goes inside...feeling coolness with the inhalation...perhaps labeling it coolness...inhaling coolness... And now, begin to notice its opposite, and how it feels warmer when breathing out... noticing warmth each time the air is naturally exhaled...feeling the warmth from deep inside on the exhalation...following the warm sensations... And now, alternating awareness between the coolness when breathing in and warmth when breathing out. Sensing the shift in temperature from coolness to warmth as your breathing continues, on and on.

[Pause]

Now, either stay with just the coolness of the inhalation or find another place somewhere on your body that feels cool...perhaps it's on your forehead...maybe it's a cool place on a hand or foot...just so it's a cool place, even cold... Take time to explore and recognize the cool sensation...be curious about the coolness...attentive to the coolness, wherever it feels cool...receptive, neither avoiding it nor holding on...just continue being aware of coolness... If you like, use your imagination to enhance the sensation of coolness, like what it feels like to be cold, really cold, like during the deep chill of winter, just for now.

[Pause]

Now, let's go with the opposite of coolness. Either go with the warm feelings of breathing out or find another place somewhere on your body that feels warm, being aware of a place that feels warm, nice and warm. Perhaps it's under your arm...maybe there's a warm place on your back...just so it's a warm place...noticing what warmth actually feels like right now, all by itself...letting the warmth be felt...fully aware of the warmth, feeling the warmth directly... If you wish, use your mind's eye to enhance the sensation of warmth, like how it feels when a blast of air rushes out when opening a hot oven door...or the hot sun beaming its heat.

[Pause]

If you like, practice alternating back and forth on your own, going between sensing the opposing sensations of coolness and the warmth. Take your time to really feel each sensation by itself, and then feeling the contrast of the other one...going back and forth by yourself...sensing coolness for a while and then sensing warmth for a while.

[Pause]

While this is happening, give yourself this opportunity to be aware of and notice the aspect of yourself that allows for switching back and forth. The piece of yourself that stays constant and Present while your experience goes through changes. It's like eavesdropping on this experience.

[Pause]

Let's try something different, that of sensing both coolness and warmth at the same time. Feeling the sensation of coolness and warmth simultaneously...sensing both the warm and the cool places together...welcoming and feeling the warm and cool places at the same time, and realizing what happens as this takes place... perceiving both coolness and warmth at the same time...and noticing this experience on your own and what's it like inside yourself while doing this... And perhaps being aware of yourself having this experience, just as it is...and maybe even stepping back and resting in pure awareness and Presence...just as it is without having to react in any way, without anything else.

[Pause]

Feel free to shift yourself around if you wish...and settle back in.

## Stage 3: Releasing Mental, Emotional, and Limiting Beliefs (Mano Maya Kosha)

Let's use this technique to explore some thoughts, emotions, and beliefs, and their opposites. If you like, use your imagination to remember a time, a place, or a circumstance when you felt perfectly calm and at ease. Perhaps it's happening now. Otherwise, a time of feeling peaceful and happy. It might come from a memory, or you can use your imagination and make it up. As long as it's a time, a place, or a circumstance of feeling calm, peaceful, and at ease. Use your senses to bring it alive more and more, using whichever senses you can to bring about feelings of being peaceful, calm, and at ease. Remembering all about it…sensing where you were…possibly how it looks…and perhaps the sounds of peace and calmness, and being content…sensing smells, noticing aromas and fragrances… Notice how all this feels in your body now. Having a direct experience in your body of feeling peaceful, calm, and totally at ease. Being aware of what peace and calm feels like right now…and experience where these feelings and sensations are now accessible in your body at this time.

Let's change gears and explore its opposite. This time, use your imagination to remember a time, a place, or a circumstance when you felt stressed out, a time of experiencing feeling nervous and tense. Let the feelings come back, just for now, and if it gets too intense, simply take a big breath in and sigh it out. Feeling stress by using your senses to bring it alive now. Using whichever senses you can to bring feelings on of being stressed and nervous, perhaps uptight. Remembering all about it…sensing where you were…how it may have looked…and sounds associated with stress and tension…perhaps sensing smells, bringing aromas back… Notice how all this feels in your body now. Having a direct experience, once again, in your body of feeling stressed, troubled, and out of sorts. And now, being passively aware of what it feels like to experience stress...and noticing where these feelings happen in your body for you. Perceiving how this expresses itself physically... observing whatever sensations are happening and wherever tension is physically being felt inside.

Okay then, take a big breath in and sigh it out. If you wish, stretch a bit and settle yourself down.

[Pause]

Let's explore the opposite of feeling stressed again. Switch back to imagining and experiencing peace, calmness, and feeling at ease all over again. Really get into it, just for now. Sensing once again what peace, calmness, and being content is like. If needed, use your memory or your imagination to spark feelings of being peaceful, calm, and perfectly at ease... You can do it. Getting back into the direct experience of feeling at ease.

[Pause]

Using your own timing, alternate back and forth between feeling stressed and feeling at ease. Take enough time to explore each of these opposites. Be curious. Getting comfortable with both. Really feeling one for a while and then moving to the other for a while. It's up to you.

[Pause]

And for now, give yourself this opportunity to sense being aware of your experience of switching back and forth. Observing...witnessing... And even taking a step back, witnessing yourself experiencing this...watching all this happen as if you were a casual observer... And getting in touch with the internal quality that stays constant and Present while your experience goes through changes.

[Pause]

If you will, give yourself a few moments to feel both opposites at the same time by making room for feeling peace and tension at the same time...physically experiencing peace and calm along with experiencing stress and tension...allowing peacefulness and tension to be experienced simultaneously...more and more aware...totally aware.

To further this experience, you can either stay with exploring the opposites of stress and peace or you can choose two more opposites. Perhaps you're ready to explore a pair of opposite qualities that are relevant to you, something that involves a feeling or an emotion or a belief. For instance, you might be interested in exploring the contrast between your sankalpa and its opposite, or maybe the opposites of clarity and confusion, or confidence and self-doubt, or a limiting thought you seem to have. For instance, you might try the belief that you're always wrong and pair it with the belief that you're always right. Whatever qualities you choose, first thoroughly explore and experience one aspect of the pair, then the other, and then change back and forth. You may even want to practice feeling the pairs simultaneously and eavesdropping on your experience.

[Pause]

### Stage 4: Cultivating Intuition (Vijnana Maya Kosha)

And as this exploration continues, awareness expands into an intuitive space, a wise space of inner knowing where creativity and intuition naturally arise...a place where insights spontaneously surface and answers are revealed. If you wish, take this opportunity for understanding to occur around an issue you're dealing with, for solutions to unanswered questions to come forth, and for messages and insights that would be helpful to you to arise.

[Pause]

## Stage 5: Experiencing Joyfulness (Ananda Maya Kosha)

You're now being invited to experience sensations of pleasure, happiness, and joy. Being more and more aware of these qualities. Inner joy is already yours and always present within. If it has become dim or hidden, it can be restored to its natural brilliance and luminosity, more and more. If it's helpful, you're invited to remember and relive experiences of joy now by recalling happy memories, smiling faces, pleasurable experiences, and peaceful times... And now, let these memories and sensations fade into deeply sensing that all is well, just as it is, and flowing into experiencing innate well-being, contentment, and blissfulness.

[Pause]

## Stage 6: Dwelling in True Nature (Atma)

When you're ready, let this all go for now by flowing and dissolving into spaciousness and boundless awareness, where it's timeless and effortless and there's infinite consciousness. Allowing yourself to be Present and being in touch with that aspect of your Self that knows and doesn't change. Residing in pure awareness.

[Long, silent pause]

# Part 4: Remembering Your Sankalpa

Om shanti—peace, peace, peace... Now, it's time to transition into remembering your sankalpa. Be consistent. Bring your sankalpa back to mind and repeat it three or so times with feeling and from your heart, allowing it to sink in deeply and meaningfully... Imagine what it would be like if it were already true.

[Pause]

## Part 5: Transition Back to Full Awareness

And now, let yourself reflect back on your experience...sensing what you've experienced...just reflecting on your experience, whatever it happened to be.

[Pause]

It's time to start transitioning back to full awareness, and to bring back all the peace, and the understanding, and the Presence you've experienced, for your sake, and for the sake of others.

Start bringing your attention back to your Presence in these surroundings, to this time and space. Sensing the ceiling above...and the walls all around... And sensing the surface below you, feeling the contact points between your body and the surface supporting you, having a direct experience of this support.

Bring your attention back to your breathing, and each time you breathe, your energy begins its steady return...your mind becomes crystal clear...feeling yourself waking up, becoming alert... When you're ready, start stretching yourself all over, waking up. Becoming more and more aware and alert... When you're ready, roll to your side for a while... To sit back up, use your arms for support to move yourself from being on your side to sitting upright...

Take a big breath in and sigh it out... Rest your hands on your knees and softly touch the tips of your thumbs to the tips of your index fingers. Close your eyes and soak it in... When your eyes open, you'll feel alert and awake, aware, and fully Present.

# Variations

Repetition of the same yoga nidra method is very valuable, so don't be too quick in trying new ones. Like most worthwhile things, this technique is likely to take time to develop and master. The point is not to get to the end of it but to actually have the desired experience. Different layers of experience will be uncovered with repetition as your needs change and your understanding develops. Let your expectations go to keep your practice fresh. Remember, it's all right to "start off slowly—and taper off."

It's also true that endless variations exist for modifying the methods used for experiencing yoga nidra. Feel free to experiment to find your preferred ways of experiencing it. Make up your own recipe by using your favorite parts from the exercises in previous chapters. When trying variations for a full practice, the best outcomes will come by keeping the five parts in place and in order. An easy way to make changes is to vary the length of time spent on each part.

- *Practice individual components.* Enjoy the benefits of individual parts and stages of the process on their own. In other words, create a practice out of just experiencing sensory awareness or autogenic training. Feel free to apply this principle to the other two yoga nidra experiences in this book.

- *Change the wording.* Substituting "the arm" for "my arm" is a change that can come after a while. This word replacement changes the experience from personally identifying with your body to one of nonattachment and witnessing the body.

- *Practice alternate-nostril breathing.* Rather than focusing your awareness on the coolness of the inhalation and the warmth of relaxation in stage 2, focus on how it feels to breathe in and out of one nostril at a time. In other words, even though you are breathing with both nostrils, focus your attention on breathing in and out of the right nostril for a while and then switch to focus on the other side. Another option is to switch back and forth from one nostril to the other—as in feeling the breath coming in on one side and going out the other. Refer to appendix 2 for more details on alternate-nostril breathing.

■ *Expand your pairs of opposites.* Refer back to your Assess Your Stress questionnaire and choose sensations, feelings, and beliefs to use for experiencing pairs of opposites during stage 3.

■ *Focus on what needs attention now.* Scan your mindbody for what is currently calling for attention in the moment and focus on it. Be aware of your experience as it naturally changes. Work with its opposite if that is helpful.

■ *Dedicate time to the chakras.* Bring your awareness to the location listed in the second column. Take your time for sensing the physical feelings and sensations associated with each pair of opposites singularly, and then in unison. The pairs in the table will get you started:

| Chakra | Location | Pairs | |
|---|---|---|---|
| Root | Base of spine, legs, feet | Safe<br>Courage<br>Worthy | Unsafe<br>Fear<br>Unworthy |
| Sacral | Pelvis, low back, abdomen | Creative<br>Sensitive<br>Awareness of needs | Stuck<br>Numb<br>Unawareness of needs |
| Solar plexus | Between the navel and heart | Confident<br>Responsible<br>Self-acceptance | Unconfident<br>Irresponsible<br>Shame/guilt |
| Heart | Heart, lungs, arms | Love/affection<br>Kindhearted<br>Forgiving | Hate/disgust<br>Hard-hearted<br>Unforgiving |

| Throat | Throat, mouth, ears, hands | Honest Self-expression Clear communication | Dishonest Repression Poor communication |
|---|---|---|---|
| Third eye | Area between the eyebrows | Knowing/ intuitive Witness awareness Trust | Confused/ uncertain Witness unawareness Distrust |
| Crown | Top of head | Belonging Feeling connected Wise/smart | Separation Feeling disconnected Unwise/foolish |

# What to Remember

- Autogenic training is a technique that is based on the mindbody connection and habituation. It brings automatic, unconscious physical reactions under control and awakens sensitivity, increases awareness, and provides stress relief.

- The awareness advantage is developed by improving concentration, mindfulness, witness consciousness, and relaxation skills. These are valuable tools for stress prevention and treatment—and most importantly, for feeling relaxed energy, inner peace, and joy.

- Deliberately and systematically experiencing opposite pairs of physical sensations, feelings, emotions, and beliefs brings about self-acceptance, harmony, and wholeness. It cultivates witness consciousness and Atma awareness.

- Lean toward balance and wholeness.

# Inner Light

The inner light is always with me.
When I slip beneath the agitated
surface of the mind, I find it,
like a fragment of the Big Bang,
still glowing. This energy doesn't
depend on health or strength
or even mental peace. It isn't a
product of belief, nor is it "me" in
any egocentric way of speaking.
The inner light is always there,
waiting to be felt and seen, waiting
for me to release it through my
choice to be still and recognize
its presence. The illumination
grows the more I let it go. Like
radiant heat it flows out of me,
flows from my whole being
without leaving me depleted.
We're all like this—whether we
know it yet or not—tiny stars,
glowing in the dark.

—Danna Faulds

*Appendix 1*

# Mudras for Supplementing
# Yoga Nidra

I was a complete skeptic when I was first introduced to *mudras*. I rolled my eyes in disbelief, even though they are known for being effective and easy to learn, practical and powerful, and available to everyone. Mudras, a Sanskrit word pronounced MOO-*drahs*, refers to yoga positions, gestures, and seals that are mostly practiced using the hands and fingers to facilitate wellness, healing, psychological balance, and spiritual transformation. Some mudras use the whole body, whereas a few others focus on just the face, particularly the eyes. As we shall see, most mudras are multipurpose in nature.

One day, my allergies and sinuses were bogging me down. Instead of taking medication, I put the *bhramara mudra* to the test. In no time at all, my nose quit running, my eyes stopped watering, and my sneezing ended. It was exciting to share my experience with others and hear how well it worked for them. Later, I discovered that the *kubera mudra* (described later) also brought relief to my sinuses. My investigation began in earnest.

A very strong relationship exists between the brain and the hands. Approximately 25 percent of the motor cortex in the brain is assigned to the hands and fingers. (Refer to the diagram of the sensory-motor cortex found in chapter 5 to see this connection.) It is believed that mudras use hand and finger positions to communicate with the brain, and then the brain communicates important signals to the rest of the body. Breathing frequency, depth, and pace are definitely influenced by holding mudras.

Mudras date back many centuries in the Yoga tradition and can be found in hatha yoga, tantra yoga, and meditation. They also have a home in India's Ayurvedic medicine, Chinese medicine, and in Jin Shin Jyutsu from Japan. The hand and finger positions held when mudras are practiced are associated with reflexology, meridians, nadis, acupressure points, and the chakras. Likewise, many religions use specific hand positions as part of their tradition. Placing the palms and fingers together in front of the heart for prayer is a good example.

Three mudras, out of the hundreds that are available, have been specially chosen to complement yoga nidra. The book *Mudras: For Healing and Transformation*, by Joseph and Lilian Le Page (2013), is highly recommended to further your understanding of mudras. They generously granted their permission to use the illustrations from their book in this one.

The arm and hand position most often recommended during yoga nidra is to have your arms away from your body with your palms up. This relieves tension in the arms and hands and creates a sense of receptiveness. Placing the fingers upward so they are not touching anything neutralizes the sensitive nerve endings in the fingertips to reduce distractions.

## Kubera Mudra

The kubera mudra is especially useful when establishing intentions and achieving goals. Use this mudra when formulating and repeating your *sankalpa* during your yoga nidra practice to give it extra energy. Try adding it to your daily meditations and while doing hatha yoga postures.

There are many benefits of the kubera mudra:

- Energy for something strongly desired becomes focused and concentrated.

- Powerful strength is put behind future plans (such as goals and whatever you want fulfilled).

- Confidence, calmness, and peacefulness are fortified.

- Energy to overcome obstacles is provided.

- Stress, worry, and resentment are reduced.

- The solar plexus (third chakra) is stimulated, which aids digestion, self-esteem, and determination.

- Finding something (e.g., a lost object, parking spot, etc.) can be aided with this mudra.

- Physically, frontal sinuses are opened and decongested. (Hold the mudra with both hands while you breathe in, sniffing the air upward as if you are smelling the fragrance of a beautiful flower; then breathe out naturally.)

## How to Do Kubera Mudra

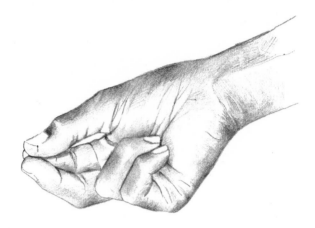

1. Touch the tip of your thumb, index finger, and middle finger together.

2. Bend the other two fingers in toward the middle of your hand so the tips touch the center of the palm.

3. Do this with both hands and rest them on your lap or out to your sides.

4. Hold for several minutes and repeat two to three times throughout the day. Focus your attention on your desired outcome.

## Hakini Mudra

Hakini mudra is quite useful during yoga nidra, as it deepens respiration naturally and influences the chakras in a positive manner. It can be held at the beginning for centering or used during the breath awareness stage. In addition, use this mudra throughout the day to enliven your breath and clear your mind. Here are some benefits of the hakini mudra:

- The breath, awareness, and energy are directed to the entire body to balance the mindbody physically and energetically.

- Complete and full breathing is facilitated effortlessly.

- Stress is reduced.

- The first six energy chakras are stimulated and harmonized.

- Both hemispheres of the brain are integrated and invigorated.

- Memory and concentration are boosted, and problem solving is assisted.

## How to Do Hakini Mudra

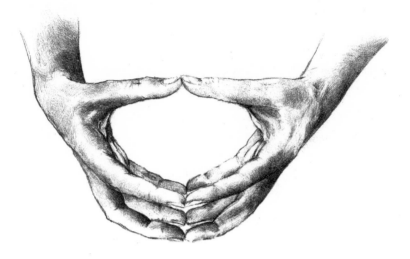

1. Gently touch the fingertips and thumb of one hand to the corresponding fingertips and thumb on the other.

2. Hold your palms apart as if you were holding a ball.

3. Place your hands in front of your solar plexus (midsection).

4. If your fingernails are too long to touch the fingertips together, interlace all the fingers, separate your palms, and touch the tips of the thumbs together.

# Ishvara Mudra

Ishvara mudra draws the senses inward to encourage *pratyahara*, the fifth limb of Raja (Ashtanga) yoga and one of the primary goals of yoga nidra. Use it whenever you feel overwhelmed with what is happening around you and for centering and calming your nerves. There are several benefits of this mudra:

- The nervous system is calmed and stress is reduced.

- Physically, circulation to the abdominal area is improved and digestion is aided.

- The need for useless sensory stimulation is reduced.

- Mental restlessness is decreased and clarity is strengthened.

- Sensory awareness is directed inward.

- Inner silence is supported, serving as a doorway to your true Self.

## How to Do Ishvara Mudra

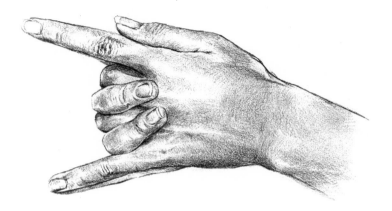

1. Interlace your fingers together.

2. Straighten the pointer and little fingers, and touch them together.

3. Gently bring the palms together.

4. Rest the extended thumbs against the index fingers.

5. Keep your shoulders back and down. Place the elbows out to your sides at the level of the abdomen with the extended fingers pointing forward.

## Mudra Meditation

Enjoy this mudra meditation as an alternative to a traditional yoga nidra practice. Begin by sitting up tall. Maintain the natural curves of your spine with your head, neck, and spine in alignment. Roll your shoulders back and down. Shake your hands like you're air-drying them.

Next, rub your hands together as if you are putting on some lotion.

Center yourself and be observant. Let your breath naturally change according to the mudra being used.

Use light finger pressure while holding mudras. If your fingers are stiff, use one hand to place the other into position. Try using your lap to prop the fingers into place. Don't give up!

1. Hold your hands in the kubera mudra on your lap. Close your eyes or let them be slightly open. Let your breathing be effortless. Be alert to the natural effects of the mudra on your mind-body and breath. Silently say your sankalpa sincerely about three times. Sit quietly for several more minutes.

2. Change your hands to the hakini mudra and hold for two to ten minutes. Gently focus your awareness on your breathing. When your mind wanders, kindly bring your attention back to your breath. Alternatively, lightly press the fingertips against each other one at a time, slowly and deliberately. In other words, press the fingertips of your little fingers together slightly, release the pressure, then press and release the ring fingertips, and so on. After touching the thumb tips together, start again with the little fingers. This will increase your focus and help balance the chakras.

3. Change your hands to the ishvara mudra to draw your senses inward. Let your mind rest and be at peace. If your mind wanders, bring your attention back to the moment. Sit quietly for several more minutes.

4. Change your hands back to the kubera mudra again while earnestly stating your sankalpa three times.

5. Finally, release your hands, open your eyes, stretch, and enjoy a smile.

## Tips for Using Yoga Mudras

To experience the full benefits of yoga mudras, consider these recommendations:

- *Integrate mudras into other activities.* Doing so reinforces the benefits of yoga nidra throughout the day. They can be added to practicing yoga postures, during meditation, while waiting in line or traffic, and during a walk.

- *Use mudras like a shield.* When practiced this way, they can counteract mental and emotional commotion.

- *Hold mudras for at least thirty seconds.* Opinions vary on how long to hold a mudra, but, in general, hold them from thirty seconds to five minutes each time. To help chronic conditions, hold them for fifteen minutes at a time, three times a day, and for three or so weeks.

- *Treat mudras like you would medicine.* Use yoga mudras on an as-needed basis, much like you would take an occasional allergy pill for relief. For long-term help and for chronic conditions, use mudras on a regular basis as described above.

- *Be smart when using mudras.* Use them to supplement appropriate medical care and to enhance your well-being.

# Breathing Options for Stress Relief and to Increase Energy (Prana)

B reathing properly improves respiration, circulation, heart health, and even digestion. It elicits the relaxation response; generates prana, the life force; and takes us right into the present moment of body awareness. Breathing fully and mindfully can free you from stress, worry, and unhappiness in that moment. This awareness gives us access to our feelings. When we truly welcome and witness feelings they fade into awareness—awareness without words. This state of awareness sets up the conditions for clear thinking and better problem solving. Likewise, the joys of daily living are readily experienced.

Practice these breathing exercises and meditations on their own, or substitute them during yoga nidra part 3, stage 2 (*prana maya kosha*). Refer to appendix 3 for more breathing exercises.

## Essential Breathing Tips

Breathe in a way that is smooth, even, and uninterrupted. Use your nose rather than your mouth to prepare the air for the lungs by filtering, warming or cooling, and moistening it. Breathe with your mouth only if necessary and to the degree needed.

Utilize your full lung capacity when you are lying down, sitting up, or standing tall. Keep the rest of your body as relaxed and free from tension as possible. Breathe down deeply so your belly moves in and out with each breath instead of only breathing into your throat or upper chest.

If you start feeling lightheaded or dizzy, your system is probably not used to this new ratio of oxygen to carbon dioxide yet. Lessen your effort until these sensations pass, then try again. Likewise, you are over-doing your exhalation if you feel the need to gasp for air.

Make sure that your abdominal muscles expand while inhaling and contract when exhaling. Watch a baby breathe to see this happen. Reverse breathing happens when the opposite takes place (the belly moves in when inhaling and out when exhaling). Reverse breathers are prone to chronic tension in the upper body, especially around the jaw, neck, upper back, and shoulders. It can contribute to mental confusion, panic, heartburn, indigestion, bloating, and gas.

Notice your breathing patterns throughout the day, and deepen it if it is shallow, rapid, or arrhythmic. Get used to breathing fully in all types of situations, especially when under stress.

## The Complete Breath

Take these steps to experience full, deep breathing:

1. First, notice how you're feeling inside using a scale of one to ten. If you're feeling extremely calm, relaxed, and peaceful, give yourself a one or two. If you're feeling extremely jittery and nervous, give yourself a nine or ten. Otherwise, give yourself a number from three to eight if you're somewhere in between feeling calm and jittery.

2. Notice how you're currently breathing. Without changing it, notice if you're breathing through your nose or mouth.

3. Take a few minutes to notice where you feel your breath going. Is it most noticeable around your nose or throat? Can you feel it entering and filling the upper chest area? Perhaps it is reach-ing all the way down into your lungs so that you feel your

abdomen rising with each inhalation and falling with each exhalation.

4. Still without making any changes, notice the pace and timing of your breathing by counting the duration of your inhalation and exhalation. Give yourself a few minutes to notice.

5. Now, gently place your hands flat against your navel. Breathing from your nose, begin lengthening your exhalation. Simply breathe out longer and slower by going beyond your typical exhalation. Don't rush; take your time. Doing so will give your body a chance to rid itself of stale, residual air and carbon dioxide. Breathing out fully also prepares your lungs for each incoming breath. Eventually, you can even compress the belly back further toward your spine. Remember to be gentle instead of forceful. Let your inhalation naturally follow each full exhalation. The inhalation will most likely be fuller since the complete exhalation has made room for more incoming air. Allow your abdominal wall to expand with each inhalation. The belly soothingly rises, making more space inside.

6. If you get distracted and notice your mind wandering, welcome to the club! Just bring your attention back to breathing. Do this as often as needed. It's good practice.

7. Next, place your hands around the sides of your rib cage. Keep the air coming in and going out abdominally as in step 5. But now, allow your rib cage to also expand while inhaling and pull back in while exhaling. Practice for several breaths.

8. Now, place one hand back down upon your navel and the other one at the level of your heart but in the center of your chest. This will remind you to breathe in deeply and fully from the bottom to the top of your lungs and back out again. Each time you breathe in and out, do so fully and slowly. Notice how you're using more of your lung capacity. Practice for several minutes.

9. Turn your attention back to the timing of your breathing. If you're breathing in for a count of four or five, begin breathing out to a count of five to ten for several minutes. Remember not to rush yourself or use force. It's important for your exhalation to become longer than your inhalation. This is how to turn off the stress reaction and turn on the relaxation response.

10. Once again, notice how you're feeling inside using a scale of one to ten. Notice any differences that were made by adjusting your breathing. If you were breathing as suggested, you should be feeling calmer and fresher, and your mind is probably clearer as well.

If you made yourself breathe in such a way that your inhalation was longer that your exhalation (for example, breathing in for five to ten and out for four), you could make yourself feel nervous and even panicky. Although not recommended, try it if you want to prove it to yourself.

During the fight-flight-freeze reaction, your breathing automatically becomes shallow and arrhythmic and thus affects how you feel. Luckily, you can control your breathing so that you can now activate the relaxation response anytime. As a valuable bonus, breathing consciously is meditative since it brings your awareness into the moment.

## The Sighing Breath

Tension is relieved by taking a big breath in through your nose and sighing it out through your mouth. Try it now, perhaps three to five times. Sighing in this manner soothes the nervous system and is calming. The problem with sighing in public is that others might ask you if something is bothering you. Therefore, it is best to practice this in private when a quick stress reliever is needed.

# Triangle Breathing

Triangle breathing brings about inner balance. It is effective for increasing your energy when feeling tired, calming your nerves when feeling anxious, and promoting sound sleep.

There are three parts to triangle breathing. The important thing is for the exhalation, inhalation, and the breath retention to be equal in duration. Therefore, adjust the rate of counting to four more quickly or more slowly depending on your lung capacity and comfort.

Part 1: Breathe out through your nose to the count of four.

Part 2: Breathe in through your nose to the count of four.

Part 3: Hold your breath to the count of four.

Repeat the whole process for a few minutes or until the desired effect happens.

# Alternate-Nostril Breathing

Alternate-nostril breathing reduces stress and creates a sense of physical, mental, and emotional well-being. This yogic breath is done by alternating nostrils while breathing. Doing so balances right- and left-brain integration and promotes mental clarity and whole brain functioning. It can relieve sinus problems and most headaches. It calms emotions and fosters feelings of deep inner contentment and balance. Due to its calming effect, it is ideal as preparation for deep relaxation or meditation.

The *nadis* (pronounced *NAH-deez*), the nonphysical nerve channels within the body, are balanced by alternate-nostril breathing. Yogis say that prana is distributed through the nadis. While there are considered to be more than 72,000 nadis that travel throughout the body, there are three primary ones that run along the spine:

- The *ida* (pronounced *EE-dah*) is just to the left of the spine and is activated by the exhalation. It is associated with receptiveness, intuition, and passivity.

- The *pingala* (pronounced *pin-GAH-lah*) is activated by the inhalation and is directly to the right of the spine. It is associated with activity, logic, and objectiveness.

- The *sushumna* (pronounced *soo-SHOOM-nah*) is the central channel and is activated by the gap between breaths. It is linked with wisdom and the balancing of our active and receptive nature.

The first step to the practice is to learn the proper hand position, or *mudra*, to aid in the alternation of the breath. Two hand positions are offered and both are effective. Try them both to find out which feels easier for you. Take a few minutes to get used to switching between nostrils with the hand positions before adding the breathing patterns.

The first way, named *Vishnu mudra*, is to take your right hand and bend your index and middle fingers to the palm. This will leave your thumb, ring, and pinkie fingers upright. Next, get used to gently closing your right nostril first with your thumb, and then release the thumb and close your left nostril with the ring finger of your right hand. Switch back and forth until it feels smooth.

*Nasagra mudra* is another hand position that can be used. Begin by making the peace sign with your right hand. Next, bring your index and middle fingers together and then release your thumb. Place the pads of your index and middle fingers in the center of your forehead or between your eyebrows and then use your thumb and the knuckle of your ring finger to alternately close and release your nostrils.

The rhythm of the inhalation to the exhalation is usually uneven at first, but it will smooth out with practice so they become equal in length. When this is easy for you, begin slowing the exhalation down so that it becomes longer than the inhalation until eventually the exhalation is about twice as long as your inhalation. Maintain alertness of your breath instead of breathing mechanically.

## Process

While either hand position can be used, the Vishnu mudra is used here to describe the pattern for the sake of clarity. The pattern alternates nostrils after each inhalation like this: Exhale, inhale; change nostril; exhale, inhale; change nostril; and so on.

Here's how to practice one round:

1.  Come into a comfortable seated position with your spine erect.

2.  Form your fingers of your right hand into the Vishnu mudra by curling your index and middle fingers into your palm, straightening the ring and little fingers. Next place your thumb against your right nostril. Rest your left hand on your left knee while touching the tips of your thumb and index finger together.

3.  Gently and slowly exhale and inhale through your left nostril.

4.  Close the left nostril with the ring finger.

5.  Release the thumb. Gently and slowly exhale and inhale through the right nostril. Close that side and return to step 3.

6.  Repeat, alternating nostrils after each inhalation. Begin practicing for two minutes and gradually, very gradually, increase to ten minutes. Avoid strain or force.

# 10 Short Relaxation, Breathing, and Meditation Options (1 to 10 Minutes)

Taking time for guided relaxation and meditation is well worth the time and effort to stay refreshed, feel energized, and focus your mind. It is important that you find ways to include these techniques into each and every day. Remember: they only work if you do them regularly!

There are times, however, when a full yoga nidra practice is not an option; shortened practices are useful in these instances. Relaxation techniques are often needed on the spot when stress strikes. Here are a variety of brief, effective techniques for your stress relief toolbox. Feel free to modify them to your liking.

## For Relaxation

### Releasing and Expanding

This relaxation exercise effectively relieves stress and revives your energy in two to ten minutes. It can be used as a substitute for relaxing physically and energetically (*anna* and *prana maya koshas*) in the preceding yoga nidra exercises. This short power nap can be done either lying on your back or sitting in a chair.

## Process

Close your eyes and begin settling down onto the floor or chair... Let yourself sink down into the surface and become more and more aware of your physical body.

All at once, stretch out and expand yourself by reaching out and tensing your arms and legs, open up your eyes wide, and stretch out your tongue. Tighten up your chest and stomach and hold it for several moments... Relax all at once by letting your whole body go loose and soft. Take a few moments to feel the relief of letting the tightness and tension leave.

Now, curl up, contract, and pull in. Pull your feet and legs in. Bend your elbows and make two fists. Compress your abdomen. Squint your eyes, purse your lips, and scrunch up your nose. Hold, hold, hold...and let go... Stretch out and take it easy.

Take in a few full, complete breaths as follows: Breathe in deeply through your nose, filling up the low, mid, and upper portion of your lungs... Open your mouth and let the air rush out. Do this a few more times.

Let your breathing return to normal, breathing through your nose...and each time you breathe out, let yourself relax more and more.

Let's mentally scan your body, while giving yourself permission to relax and let go of muscular tension even further.

Become aware of your toes and feet and allow them to soften and relax...and feel the softening spreading to your calves and on up to your hips. Allow any tightness or tension remaining in the lower body to roll down your legs and safely away.

Now your lower back is relaxing...mid-back...upper back, and the shoulders are all letting go of muscular tension... Allow your upper arms to relax…your elbows…your forearms…your hands and your fingers. Allow any tension remaining in the upper body to roll down your arms and safely away… Everything's relaxing, more and more.

Allow your torso and vital organs in your abdomen to be at ease… And now, all around your ribs are softening and relaxing…front… back…and sides, at ease.

Feel your neck and throat relax…all the muscles in your face are relaxing too. Your mouth…tongue…nose…your cheeks…eyes and forehead are very relaxed.

The feeling of relaxation flows from the top of your head all the way back down to your toes, like a refreshing waterfall. Feel yourself becoming even more relaxed.

At the count of three, you can feel even more relaxed and at ease. One, relaxing more…two, more and more…and three, just right.

When you're ready, begin to stretch and move gently. Open your eyes and you'll feel calm, relaxed, and rested.

Smile.

## Easy Does It

Try this five-minute technique if you are especially tired. Since it doesn't involve tensing your muscles prior to relaxing them, it's particularly helpful if you have physical conditions such as arthritis, fibromyalgia, or other difficulties with tensing your muscles. Easy Does It incorporates physical, energetic, and mental relaxation, as well as intuition. During it, an inner sanctuary of peace and calm is developed using guided imagery. The sanctuary can be recalled and experienced during stressful times to bring relief or during yoga nidra if it gets too intense and a break is needed.

## Process

If possible, kick your shoes off, put your feet up, and uncross your legs and arms. Let yourself sink comfortably into a chair (or the floor). Close your eyes or keep them slightly open.

Begin using your breathing to create a relaxing experience... Slowly, breathe all the way in...and all the way out... Each time you breathe out, begin releasing any tightness or tenseness you may have... Tightness may be in the form of physical tension, mental confusion, or emotional distress... Just let it all clear away, each time you exhale...like clouds disappearing.

Now, take your attention to your feet... Take a nice, big breath in...and feel them softening and relaxing each time you breathe out...slowly and easily.

The next time you breathe in, let your awareness fill your legs...and when slowly breathing out, allow your calves, your knees, and your thighs to continue releasing and relaxing, each time you breathe out...and let go.

Wrap your awareness around your hips... Breathe in deeply...and feeling them soften as you breathe out...sinking and settling down, slowly and easily.

Float your attention to your back... Breathe in, and as you breathe out feel the tension in your back dissolve, letting go more and more, each time you breathe out.

Surround your shoulders with your awareness like a comforting cloak... Breathe in, and feel them softening as you breathe out... releasing the tightness and the soreness...soothing your shoulders with your slow and easy breathing.

Let this relaxed feeling begin flowing down around your shoulders, soothing your arms and hands with peace and quiet.

Become aware of your mouth… Unclench the teeth… Let the lips part slightly. As you continue breathing gently and softly, let the nose and cheeks smooth out…and allowing the eyes and forehead to soften.

Imagine letting your pores open up and breathe, feeling yourself releasing and expanding.

As you relax deeper and deeper, the peacefulness brings to mind a quiet, personal sanctuary…an extremely comfortable and safe place where you can feel surrounded with exactly what you need. Bring it alive by using all your senses.

This is a special place to feel protected and safe and understood… where you can spend some time getting to know the real you…the person you were meant to be…and feeling safe to be who you really are…and fully capable of finding answers to your questions… Treat yourself to some time to explore this special feeling and space.

After a while, allow your attention to come back to your breath… feeling more wholesome and real, and feeling your energy improving with each breath.

And, whenever you're ready, begin to stretch your body, wiggle your fingers and toes…and open your eyes…feeling refreshed and renewed.

## Quick and Easy Breathing Meditations

### Take a Breather

This breathing meditation is done to the rhythm of your inhalation and exhalation to the word "breather." Be sure to let the rate of your breathing naturally slow down to get the maximum benefit. For instance, breathe in through your nose to the count of four or five and breathe out for five to ten. Lengthening your exhalation has an extremely positive benefit because it activates the relaxation response and soothes your nervous system. It's also good for your heart.

**Process**

Breathe in **B**alance.

Breathe out **R**elief.

Breathe in **E**nergy.

Breathe out **A**ppreciation.

Breathe in **T**rust.

Breathe out **H**ope and **H**appiness.

Breathe in **E**asily.

Breathe out and **R**elax.

Repeat from the start.

## Breathing with Your Name

Choose a positive quality that begins with each letter in your name. The example below is for someone named Chris. One nice option for silently saying "I am" is to substitute "I am grateful for being [quality]" or "My true nature is [quality]." Another variation is to repeat each affirmation at your own pace rather than to the rhythm of your breath.

**Process**

Breathe in and silently say, "I am."
Breathe out and say, "Courageous."

Breathe in and silently say, "I am."
Breathe out and say, "Humorous."

Breathe in and silently say, "I am."
Breathe out and say, "Relaxed."

Breathe in and silently say, "I am."
Breathe out and say, "Intelligent."

Breathe in and silently say, "I am."
Breathe out and say, "Strong."

# Reinforcing Your Sankalpa and Awakening Your True Nature

## Breathing Life into Your Sankalpa

Clear your mind and freshen your spirit with this easy breathing technique. Use it to reinforce your sankalpa by substituting it for the one given. The *kubera mudra,* pictured in appendix 1, is used for reinforcement.

While it may be difficult to stay focused at first, it gets easier and more effective with regular practice. Feel free to spend one to ten minutes (or more) on the experience.

## Process

Sit comfortably and begin clearing your mind by focusing on the present moment. Simply settle into your chair (or floor if you're lying down)... Touch your thumbs to the index and middle fingers on the same hand while folding your ring and little finger in toward the palm. Rest your hands on your lap (or out to your sides).

Listen to the sounds around you...feel the air on your skin...notice what mood you're in. Don't even bother naming your mood. Instead, impartially notice how it feels.

Again and again, allow yourself to forget about the past and let go of the future, to stay focused upon each and every present moment. Each time you notice your attention being pulled to either the past or future, kindly focus your attention on the present moment and come back to your senses. Continue this for a few minutes.

Breathe in and silently say to yourself, "I am."

Breathe out and silently say, "Healthy and happy."

Breathe in and silently say, "I am."

Breathe out and silently say, "Healthy and happy."

Continue on for as long as desired. As soon as you notice that you've become distracted, simply let the distraction go and gently bring your attention back to your breath and your saying. If something persistently arises, it may be something that needs your attention, so take some time for discovery and exploration. The more you practice, the longer you'll be able to stay focused. As a bonus, your ability to concentrate in general will improve as well.

## Cultivate the Positive: Pratipaksha Bhavana

*Pratipaksha bhavana* (pronounced *prah-TEE-pak-shah BHAH-vah-nah*) is a meditation practice based on a teaching from Yoga Sutra II.33 that says, "When disturbed by negative thoughts and feelings, cultivate the positive" (Lusk 2005b, 179).

Although it's important to get to know all the emotions, even those that seem unpleasant or negative, it's quite important to nourish, water, and feed what you want to grow. This meditation teaches us to exchange negative thoughts and feelings for positive ones. We do this by breathing in *and* out the positive to counteract the negative.

Helpful qualities are emphasized so that they take root quickly and efficiently. The neuroplasticity of the brain, as described in chapter 3, will facilitate making positive changes that are lasting. This nurtures our capacity to react constructively and mindfully in a levelheaded and calm manner to stressful people and situations—and less likely to react automatically or negatively.

Instead of trying to be patient now, courageous tomorrow, and calm after that, choose one quality wisely and stick with it. This brings us focus rather than having to "be everything" and having to keep it all straight. If patience is chosen, for example, other qualities will naturally and automatically follow. When being patient, we are more understanding, loving, generous, kind, forgiving, and more.

Another application of pratipaksha bhavana is to literally change one's thought, feeling, or action for another. When someone is unkind and behaves badly, or when you're tempted to be critical, focus on taking positive action instead. It's similar to the carpenter who drives out the old nail with a new one.

Once you've selected a positive quality, it will no longer be necessary to think of its negative counterpart during the meditation—simply cultivate the positive. Recognize and explore when shadow thoughts and emotions naturally come up, take a step back, and ultimately let go.

## Process

Sit up tall with your head, neck, and spine aligned. Relax your shoulders back and down. Rest your hands in your lap and use the kubera mudra (see appendix 1).

Spend some time focusing your attention on your ongoing and natural breath. You may wish to say silently to yourself, "I know I'm breathing in" on the inhalation, and "I know I'm breathing out" on the exhalation. Take your time with this process of winding down. As your mind begins to wander, kindly bring your awareness back to breathing.

Choose a negative thought or feeling that you would like to transform into something positive. Possibilities include worry, fear, sadness, or being critical. What you want to work with is up to you. Choose something now that is bothersome to you.

Pause for a few moments.

Instead of holding on to the negative, or trying to push it away…let it go…set it free…let it melt away like honey in hot tea…let it evaporate like fog as the sun starts to shine.

Next, bring to mind what its positive counterpart is. For example, you could exchange clarity for worry, happiness for sadness, or understanding for being critical. Wait until you have your positive quality.

Bring your attention back to your breath. While breathing in you may say, "Breathing in, I am [name the new quality]. Breathing out, I am [name the quality]." Continue for a while.

Now, call to mind something that reminds you of the trait you're developing and nurturing. This could be a person, a place, an object, or image. Focus your attention on it, dwelling in the memory or experience of it. Take some time for this.

Look out for when your attention wanders, make room to explore the shadows with curiosity, let go, and bring your attention back to your quality and return to cultivating the positive.

To strengthen your experience, see or sense yourself in a situation or circumstance responding with the new characteristic you're cultivating. Take some time for this.

Once again, return your attention to the positive quality and welcome it inward. Remember and reflect on the positive often. When you're ready, open your eyes and stretch.

## Breathing Affirmations to Awaken Your True Nature

This exercise uses three key words for focusing and as a reminder of your true nature. Pick your favorite word and repeat each phrase three to five times each. If you prefer, substitute different positive and uplifting qualities for the ones given.

Feel free to create a positive word or phrase of your own, such as your sankalpa, and choose a characteristic for each letter in the word. If you prefer, say the affirmations at your own pace, breathing naturally, instead of timing them with your breathing. Reflect on each quality using memories, impressions, images, and so forth.

**Process**

## ATMA

Breathe in and silently say, "I am."
Breathe out and silently say, "**Alert.**"

Breathe in and silently say, "I am."
Breathe out and silently say, "**Timeless.**"

Breathe in and silently say, "I am."
Breathe out and silently say, "**Mindful.**"

Breathe in and silently say, "I am."
Breathe out and silently say, "**Aware.**"

## TRUE

Breathe in and silently say, "My true nature is."
Breathe out and silently say, "**Transcendental.**"

Breathe in and silently say, "My true nature is."
Breathe out and silently say, "**Relaxed.**"

Breathe in and silently say, "My true nature is."
Breathe out and silently say, "**Understanding.**"

Breathe in and silently say, "My true nature is."
Breathe out and silently say, "**Eternal Energy.**"

## NATURE

Breathe in and silently say, "My true nature is."
Breathe out and silently say, "Natural."

Breathe in and silently say, "My true nature is."
Breathe out and silently say, "Awareness."

Breathe in and silently say, "My true nature is."
Breathe out and silently say, "Trusting."

Breathe in and silently say, "My true nature is."
Breathe out and silently say, "Universal."

Breathe in and silently say, "My true nature is."
Breathe out and silently say, "Real."

Breathe in and silently say, "My true nature is."
Breathe out and silently say, "Energy."

# Mindfulness in a Minute

## Take 5 to Thrive

Practice every instruction for one minute each. Each time your mind wanders off, return your attention to the moment.

---

### Process

1. Stretch your arms, legs, back, and everything else.

2. Sit up tall. Roll your shoulders back and down. Rest your hands on your lap. Use the yoga hand mudra of your choice or simply rest and relax your fingers. Uncross your legs. Place your feet flat on the floor. Be still.

3. Close your eyes. Notice sounds and smells. Let each come and go without naming or judging.

4. Enjoy breathing slowly, smoothly, and deeply.

5. Open your eyes. Stretch. Feel refreshed, renewed, and ready. Smile.

---

# B...R...E...A...T...H...E for Mindfulness

This meditation provides seven steps for practicing mindfulness. The word "breathe" will help you remember each step. Take your time to fully experience each of the steps before going on to the next.

---

**Process**

Breathe fully, slowly.

Release muscular tension.

Engage and Expand your awareness.

Alert to sounds, sights, and smells—Awareness without naming.

Thoughtful, welcoming, and impartial.

Here and now.

Enjoy the moment.

---

## Stop–Look–Listen–Smile

Here's a mini-meditation that can be done anytime and anywhere. It will settle your mind down and clear your head, and your awareness will increase.

**Process**

**Stop.** Notice your posture...breath...energy level...mood...mental activity.

**Look.** Blink your eyes several times. Look at something far away and discover the details in what you see. Blink again. Look at something close up. Discover the details. Blink again. Use peripheral vision and soften your gaze.

**Listen.** Listen to sounds come and go. Simply observe without naming or judging. No resistance. No clinging.

**Smile.**

# Appendix 4

# How to Lead Others in Yoga Nidra

Here are some tips to help you lead clients, students, and friends through yoga nidra effectively. Working with yoga nidra is powerful, and it is up to you to use this book responsibly and ethically. Leaders with little or no training in yoga nidra can use these scripts with emotionally healthy people. Make sure to read through the script and practice it on your own first. Be careful, however, when presenting themes and techniques that are unfamiliar to you.

If your group is composed of people who are emotionally ill or especially fragile, seek out special training or professional guidance before introducing them to this work.

## Preparing the Group or Individual

Before beginning any guided yoga nidra exercise, describe the process and answer questions. Let participants know that if they become uncomfortable at any time, they may tune out for a while, open their eyes, and/or shift their attention to something else.

Optimally, guide others through the entire experience. If time is short, or certain parts are of particular usefulness, incorporate time for getting into the proper frame of mind by relaxing first, since it reduces anxiety, activates the mindbody connection, and enhances the ability to focus on the guided meditation. Consider incorporating relaxed breathing, since it is essential for complete and total relaxation.

Unfortunately, very few people take full breaths, especially when under stress. When a person consciously uses deep breathing correctly, stress is reduced and the mind can remain calm and stable. Remember to bring them back to full wakefulness at the end.

As you read a script, people will follow you for a while and then drift off into their own imaginations and experiences. They will usually tune back in later on. If they know this in advance, they won't feel as if they are failing by being inattentive. So tell them that this is normal and to let it happen.

When you're leading yoga nidra meditations, stay in your conscious (alert and efficient) mind. Keep your eyes open. Pay careful attention to all participants. You may have to repeat an instruction if you see that people are not following you.

## Choosing the Right Atmosphere

Select a room that has comfortable chairs for sitting or a carpeted floor for lying down. Make sure to close the door, shut the windows, and draw the blinds to block out interruptions.

If possible, find a room that has lights you can dim. Low lights enhance the ability to relax by blocking out visual distractions. If the lights cannot be controlled to your satisfaction, bring along a lamp or night lights.

Seek out a room that has its own thermostat so that you can adjust the temperature, making it warm and comfortable. If the room is too cool, it will be hard to relax and remain focused. Suggest that people wear a sweater or jacket if they think they may get cold.

If distractions occur—a noisy air conditioner, outside traffic, loud conversations from an adjoining room—try raising your voice, using shorter phrases and fewer pauses, or incorporating the sounds into the guided meditation. For example, you might say, "Notice how the humming sounds of the air conditioner relax you more and more," or "If your mind begins to drift, gently bring it back to the sound of my voice."

## Using Your Voice

Speak in a calm, comforting, and steady manner. Let your voice flow. Your voice should be smooth and somewhat monotonous. Do not whisper.

Start with your voice at a volume that can be easily heard. As the guided meditation progresses and as the participants' awareness increases, you may begin speaking more softly. As a person relaxes, hearing acuity can increase. Bring your voice up in tone when suggesting tension and bring it down when suggesting relaxation. Near the end of the guided meditation, return to using an easily heard volume to help participants come back to normal wakefulness.

Tell participants to use a hand signal if they cannot hear you. Advise people with hearing problems to sit close to you. Another option is to move closer to them.

## Pacing Yourself

Read the yoga nidra scripts slowly—but not so slowly that you lose people. Begin at a conversational pace and slow down as the relaxation progresses. It's easy to go too fast, so take your time. Don't rush.

Leader's notes and script divisions are printed as headings or in brackets and should not be read out loud. The ellipses (...) and the spaces between paragraphs indicate a brief pause. When you see [Pause], wait a little longer.

Give participants time to follow your instructions. If you suggest that they wiggle their toes, watch them do so, then wait for them to stop wiggling their toes before going on. When participants are relaxed and engaged in the yoga nidra process, they have tapped in to their subconscious mind, which operates slowly and is primed and ready for imagery—and they shouldn't be hurried.

To help you with your volume, tone, pace, and timing, listen to a recording of yourself leading the yoga nidra meditations.

As you reach the end of a meditation, always help participants make the transition back to the present. Have them sense their surroundings, stretch, and breathe deeply. Repeat these instructions until everyone is alert.

## Using Music

Using music to enhance relaxation is not a new idea. History is full of examples of medicine men and women, philosophers, ministers, scientists, and musicians who use music to heal. In fact, music seems to be an avenue of communication for some people where no other avenues appear to exist.

If you use music, it should be cued up and ready to go at the right volume before starting. Adjust the volume so that it doesn't drown out your voice. On the other hand, music that is too soft may cause listeners to strain to hear it. Nothing ruins the atmosphere more quickly than the leader having to fool around trying to get the music going.

Jim Borling, a board certified music therapist, makes the following suggestions on selecting music:

- Custom select music for individual clients or classes whenever possible. Not everyone responds in a similar fashion to the same music.

- Matching a person's present emotional state with music is known as the ISO principle. If you can match the initial state and then gradually begin changing the music, the person's emotional state will change along with the music. If a person is agitated or angry, begin with faster-paced music, then change to slower-paced selections as relaxation deepens.

- Don't assume that the type of music you find relaxing will be relaxing to others. Have a variety of musical styles available, and ask your clients for suggestions.

- Choose music that has flowing melodies rather than disjointed and fragmented melodies. Try using sounds from nature like ocean waves. Experiment with New Age music and Space music, much of which is appropriate for relaxation work. Classical music may be effective, especially movements that are marked "largo" or "adagio."

- Select music based upon the mood desired. Sedative music is soothing and produces a contemplative mood. Stimulating music increases bodily energy and stimulates the emotions. Select music with a slow tempo and low pitch. The higher the pitch or frequency of sound, the more likely it will be irritating.

## Working with Guided Imagery Meditations

Everyone is different, so each person will experience guided imagery meditations uniquely. These individual differences should be encouraged. During guided imagery, some people will imagine vivid scenes, colors, images, or sounds, while others will focus on what they are feeling, or experience it as a concept. This is why a combination of sights, sounds, and feelings have been incorporated into the meditations.

With practice, it is possible to expand your participants' range of awareness. By careful selection and use of images, you can help deepen their experience and cultivate their awareness in new areas that can enrich their lives. For instance, a person who is most comfortable in the visual area can be encouraged to stretch his or her awareness and increase his or her sensitivity to feelings and sounds.

## Processing the Experience

You may wish to add to the richness of the yoga nidra meditations by asking participants afterward to share their experiences with others. This can be facilitated by creating an atmosphere of trust. Ask the individual or group open-ended questions that relate to the theme of the exercise. Be accepting and empathetic toward everyone. Since people respond in a variety of ways to guided meditations and visualizations, avoid generalizing about the expectations and benefits of any given script. Respect everyone's comments, and never be judgmental or critical, even if people express negative reactions.

## Understanding Cautions

Do not force people to participate in anything that may be uncomfortable for them. Give ample permission to everyone to only do things that feel safe. Tell them that if something seems threatening they can change it to something that feels right, or they can stop the yoga nidra process, stretch, and open their eyes. Emphasize to participants that they are in total control, and able to leave their image-filled subconscious mind and return to their alert rational conscious mind at any time they choose. In another vein, clients may want to explore what feels uncomfortable to them in the safety of the experience.

Advise participants that it is not safe to practice meditation or visualization while driving or operating machinery.

# References and Resources

Adhana, R., R. Gupta, J. Dvivedii, et al. 2013. "The Influence of the 2:1 Yogic Breathing Technique on Essential Hypertension." *Indian Journal of Physiology and Pharmacology* 57: 38–44. http://www.ncbi.nlm.nih.gov/pubmed/24020097.

Alfonso, R. F., H. Hachul, E. H. Kozasa, et al. 2012. "Yoga Decreases Insomnia in Postmenopausal Women: A Randomized Clinical Trial." *Menopause* 19: 186–193. http://www.ncbi.nlm.nih.gov/pubmed/22048261.

American Psychological Association [APA]. "Understanding Chronic Stress." Accessed on December 17, 2014, retrieved from http://www.apa.org/help center/understanding-chronic-stress.aspx.

———. 2013. *Stress in America: Missing the Health Care Connection.* February 7. https://www.apa.org/news/press/releases/stress/2012/full-report.pdf.

Amita, S., S. Prabhakar, I. Manoj, et al. 2009. "Effect of Yoga Nidra on Blood Glucose Level in Diabetic Patients." *Indian Journal of Physiological and Pharmacology* 53 (1): 97–101.

Benson, Herbert, and William Proctor. 2010. *Relaxation Revolution: Enhancing Your Personal Health Through the Science and Genetics of Mind Body Healing.* New York: Scribner.

Borysenko, Joan. 1994. *Pocketful of Miracles: Prayer, Meditations, and Affirmations to Nurture Your Spirit Every Day of the Year.* New York: Warner Books.

Collingwood, J. 2007. "The Physical Effects of Long-Term Stress." *PsychCentral.* Retrieved on December 17, 2014, from http://psychcentral.com/lib/the -physical-effects-of-long-term-stress/000935.

Desikachar, T. K. V. 1995. *The Heart of Yoga: Developing a Personal Practice.* Rochester, VT: Inner Traditions International.

Devi, Nischala Joy. 2000. *The Healing Path of Yoga: Alleviate Stress, Open Your Heart, and Enrich Your Life.* New York: Three Rivers Press.

———. 2007. *The Secret Power of Yoga: A Woman's Guide to the Heart and Spirit of the Yoga Sutras.* New York: Three Rivers Press.

Doidge, Norman. 2007. *The Brain That Changes Itself: Stories of Personal Triumph from the Frontiers of Brain Science*. New York: Penguin.

Durgananda, Swami. 2002. *The Heart of Meditation: Pathways to a Deeper Experience*. South Fallsburg, NY: SYDA Foundation.

Easwaran, Eknath. 1987. *The Upanishads*. Tomales, CA: Nilgiri Press.

Faulds, Danna. 2004. *Prayers to the Infinite: New Yoga Poems*. Greenville, VA: Peaceable Kingdom Books.

———. 2013. *Breath of Joy: Poems, Prayers, and Prose*. Greenville, VA: Peaceable Kingdom Books.

Feuerstein, Georg. 1997. *The Shambhala Encyclopedia of Yoga*. Boston: Shambhala.

Folan, Lilias. 2005. *Lilias! Yoga Gets Better with Age*. Emmaus, PA: Rodale Press.

Goel, Arun. 2001. "Understanding Deep Relaxation Through Yoga Nidra." Accessed December 15, 2014. http://www.healthandyoga.com/html/news/nidra.aspx.

Gothe, Neha, M. B. Pontifex, C. Jillman, et al. 2013. "The Acute Effects of Yoga on Executive Function." *Journal of Physical Activity and Health* June 5.

Grøntved, Anders, A. Pan, R. A. Mckary, et al. 2014. "Muscle-Strengthening and Conditioning Activities and Risk of Type 2 Diabetes: A Prospective Study in Two Cohorts of US Women." *PLOS Medicine* 11 (1, January): e100158.

Hirschi, Gertrud. 2000. *Mudras: Yoga in Your Hands*. San Francisco, CA: Weiser Books.

Hagelin, John. 1998. "Stress Prevention: Its Impact on Health and Medical Savings." *Institute of Science Technology and Public Policy*. Congressional Prevention Coalition.

Kiecolt-Glaser, Janice, J. M. Bennett, R. Andridge, et al. 2014. "Yoga's Impact on Inflammation, Mood, and Fatigue in Breast Cancer Survivors: A Randomized Controlled Trial." *Journal of Clinical Oncology* January 27: JCO.2013.51.8860.

Krishna, B. H., P. Pal, G. K. Pal, et al. 2014. "Effect of Yoga Therapy on Heart Rate, Blood Pressure, and Cardiac Autonomic Function in Heart Failure." *Journal of Clinical and Diagnosis Research* 8: 14–16. http://www.ncbi.nlm.nih.gov/pubmed/24596712.

Krugers, H. J., C. C. Hoogenraad C. C., and L. Groc. (2010). "Stress Hormones and AMPA Receptor Trafficking in Synaptic Plasticity and Memory." *Nature Reviews Neuroscience* 11 (October): 675–681. doi:10.1038/nrn2913.

Kuchinskas, Susan. 2008. "Why Multitasking Is a Myth." *WebMD the Magazine*, http://www.webmd.com/mental-health/features/why-multitasking-isnt-efficient.

Kumar, Kamakhya. 2004. "A Study on the Impact on Stress & Anxiety Through Yoga Nidra." *Yoga Mimamsa* 36 (3): 163–69. Lonavala, Maharashtra: Kaivalyadham.

———. 2004. "Yoga Nidra and Its Impact on Students' Well-being." *Yoga Mimamsa* 36 (1): 31–35. Lonavala, Maharashtra: Kaivalyadham.

———. 2005a. "Origin and Application of Yoga Nidra." *Nature & Wealth* IV (4, October).

———. 2005b. "Effect of Yoga Nidra on Hypertension and Other Psychological Co-Relates." *Yoga the Science* 3 (7).

———. 2006. "A Study of the Improvement of Physical Mental Health Through Yoga Nidra." *Dev Sanskriti Inter-disciplinary Research Journal* 4 (4): 39–46.

———. 2007a. "The Healing Sleep." *Yoga Magazine (Body Mind Spirit)*, issue 50.

———. 2007b. "Yoga Nidra and Its Impact on Blood Cells." Souvenir of National Yoga Week, organized by Morarji Desai National Institute of Yoga, New Delhi.

———. 2008a. "A Holistic Approach to Stress Management." *Nature & Wealth* VII (4).

———. 2008b. "A Study on the Impact on Stress and Anxiety Through Yoga Nidra." *Indian Journal of Traditional Knowledge, NISCAIR New Delhi* 7(3): 405–409.

_____ 2008c. "Complete the Course of Sleep Through Yoga Nidra." *Nature & Wealth* VII (1, January).

———. 2009. "Reversing the Ischemic Heart Diseases through Yoga Nidra." *Nature & Wealth* VIII (1).

———. 2010. "Reversing the Ischemic Heart Disease Through Yogic Relaxation." Souvenir of National Yoga Week, organized by Morarji Desai National Institute of Yoga, New Delhi.

———. 2010. "Psychological Changes as Related to Yoga Nidra." *International Journal of Psychology: A Biopsychosocial Approach* 6: 129–137.

———. 2010. "Stress-Free Life Through Yoga Nidra." Souvenir, International Symposium on Yogism 36–38.

———. 2012. "A study on the Impact on ESR Level Through Yogic Relaxation Technique Yoga Nidra." *Indian Journal of Traditional Knowledge; N I S C A I R* 11 (2, April): 358–61.

———. 2013a. *A Handbook of Yoga Nidra*. New Delhi, India: D.K. Printworld.

———. 2013b. "Manage the Psycho-Complexities Through Yoga Nidra." Proceedings of National Conference on Yoga Therapy, organized at Manglore University. 18–19.

Kumar, Kamakhya, and B. Joshi. 2009. "Study on the Effect of Pranakarshan Pranayama & Yoga Nidra on Alpha EEG & GSR." *Indian Journal of Traditional Knowledge; N I S C A I R*, New Delhi 8 (3): 453–454.

Le Page, Joseph, and Lilian Le Page. 2013. *Mudras: For Healing and Transformation.* Sebastopol, CA: Integrative Yoga Therapy.

Levine, Peter. 1997. *Waking the Tiger.* Berkeley, CA: North Atlantic Books.

Loh, K.K., and R. Kanai. 2014. "Higher Media Multi-Tasking Activity Is Associated with Smaller Gray-Matter Density in the Anterior Cingulate Cortex." *PLoS One*, September 24; 9(9): e106698. doi: 10.1371/journal .pone.0106698.

Lusk, Julie. 1998. *Desktop Yoga.* New York: Penguin Putnam Inc.

———. 2004. *Wholesome Energizers CD/MP3 with Cultivate the Positive.* Milford, OH: Wholesome Resources.

———. 2005a. *Complete Chakra Chart.* Milford, OH: Wholesome Resources.

———. 2005b. *Yoga Meditations: Timeless Mind-Body Practices for Awakening.* Duluth, MN: Whole Person Associates.

———. 2006. *Power of Presence CD/MP3 with Cultivate the Positive.* Milford, OH: Wholesome Resources.

———. 2006. *Wholesome Relaxation CD/MP3 with Cultivate the Positive.* Milford, OH: Wholesome Resources.

———. 2009. *Real Relaxation: Yoga Nidra CD/MP3.* Milford, OH: Wholesome Resources.

———. 2015. *30 Scripts for Relaxation, Imagery & Inner Healing, Volume 1.* Duluth, MN: Whole Person Associates.

———. 2015. *30 Scripts for Relaxation, Imagery & Inner Healing, Volume 2.* Duluth, MN: Whole Person Associates.

———. 2015. *Relax: Yoga Nidra for Deep Relaxation for Unshakable Peace and Joy CD/MP3.* Milford, OH: Wholesome Resources.

———. 2015. *Reflect: Yoga Nidra for Sensing Inner Strength and Balance CD/MP3.* Milford, OH: Wholesome Resources.

———. 2015. *Revitalization: Yoga Nidra for High-Level Living CD/MP3.* Milford, OH: Wholesome Resources.

Mascaro, Juan. 1965. *The Upanishads.* New York: Penguin.

Mayo Clinic. 2013. "Chronic Stress Puts Your Health at Risk." July 11. Retrieved on December 17, 2014, from http://www.mayoclinic.org/healthy-living/stress -management/in-depth/stress/art-20046037.

McGonigal, Kelly. 2010–2011. "Inspired Intention: The Nature of Sankalpa." *Yoga International* Winter: 44.

Merrill, Douglas. 2012. "Why Multitasking Doesn't Work." *Forbes*, August 17, http://www.forbes.com/sites/douglasmerrill/2012/08/17/why-multitasking -doesnt-work/.

Miller, Richard. 2005. *Yoga Nidra: The Meditative Heart of Yoga*. Boulder, CO: Sounds True.

————. 2015. *The iRest Program for Healing PTSD: A Proven-Effective Approach to Using Yoga Nidra Meditation and Deep Relaxation Techniques to Overcome Trauma*. Oakland, CA: New Harbinger Publications.

————. 2015. 42 audio recordings of practices from the book *The iRest Program for Healing PTSD*. http://www.irest.us.

Mitchell, Stephen. 2000. *Bhagavad Gita: A New Translation*. New York: Harmony Books.

Muktibodhananda, Swami. 1993. *Hatha Yoga Pradipika*. Munger, Bihar, India: Bihar School of Yoga.

Naparstek, Belleruth. 1994. *Staying Well with Guided Imagery*. New York: Warner Books, Inc.

Panda, N. C. 2003. *Yoga-Nidra: Yogic Trance Theory, Practice, and Applications*. New Delhi, India: D.K. Printworld (P) Ltd.

Pandya, P., and K. Kumar. 2007. "Yoga Nidra & Its Impact on Human Physiology." *Yoga Vijnan, M.D.N.I.Y* 1(1): 1–8.

Rani, K., S. Tiwari, U. Singh, G. Agrawal, A. Ghildiyal, and N. Srivastava. 2011. "Impact of Yoga Nidra on Psychological General Wellbeing in Patients with Menstrual Irregularities: A randomized controlled trial." *International Journal of Yoga*, January–June, 4(1): 20–25.

Rosch, P.J. (Ed.). 2001. "The Quandary of Job Stress Compensation." *Health and Stress* 3:1–4.

Saraswati, Swami Satyananda. 1998. *Yoga Nidra*. Munger, Bihar, India: Yoga Publications Trust.

Satchidananda, Sri Swami. 1978. *The Yoga Sutras of Patanjali*. Yogaville, VA: Integral Yoga Publications.

————. 1988. *The Living Gita: The Complete Bhagavad Gita and Commentary*. New York: An Owl Book, Henry Holt and Company.

Scaer, Robert. 2014. *The Body Bears the Burden*. London: Routledge.

Shearer, Alistair. 1982. *The Yoga Sutras of Patanjali*. New York: Bell Tower.

Shearer, Alistair, and Peter Russell. 1978. *The Upanishads*. New York: Bell Tower.

Stetter, Friedhelm, and Sirko Kupper. 2002. "Autogenic Training: A Meta-Analysis of Clinical Outcome Studies." *Applied Psychophysiology and Biofeedback* 27, (1): 45–98.

Sodhi, C. 2014. "Assessment of the Quality of Life in Patients with Bronchial Asthma, Before and After Yoga: A Randomized Trial." *Iranian Journal of Allergy, Asthma, and Immunology* 13: 55–60. http://www.ncbi.nlm.nih.gov /pubmed/24338229.

Talbot, Shawn. 2011. *The Cortisol Connection: Why Stress Makes You Fat and Ruins Your Health—And What You Can Do About It.* Alameda, CA: Hunter House.

Taylor, S. E., L. C. Klein, B. P. Lewis, et al. 2000. "Biobehavioral Responses to Stress in Females: Tend-and-Befriend, Not Fight-or-Flight." *Psychological Review* 107: 441–429.

Weintraub, Amy. 2004. *Yoga for Depression: A Compassionate Guide to Relieve Suffering Through Yoga.* New York: Broadway Books.

———. 2012. *Yoga Skills for Therapists: Effective Practices for Mood Management.* New York: Norton.

# Additional Resources

Visit **Wholesome Resources** (http://wholesomeresources.com) for additional books, articles, recordings, research, and trainings from Julie Lusk and other experts on yoga, yoga nidra, meditation, guided imagery, stress management, and relaxation. Join our community by telling your stories, asking your questions, and sharing your answers with us.

## This Is What I Have to Say to You

This is what I have to say to you. Enter the center of
your being. Stand in the source of all inquiry,
knowing, and unknowing.
Reclaim your wholeness by being the body and all
its changing sensations. Receive the message of
your emotions without believing they're the only
show in town. Be the subtle energy that ebbs and
flows, that brings healing and connection. Be the
mind, witnessing thoughts, sinking into insight and
unleashed creativity. Be the innate bliss and joy
that arises when no part of you is exiled or left to
fester in darkness.
At the center, be the conscious self without borders
or limits. Slip outside personal identity to find that
the infinite reality of truth has always been you.
From the center of the center, let what you are
express freely on all levels. Present, awake, and
grateful for this moment, just be, without qualifiers
or boundaries, and in the being, be at peace.

—Danna Faulds

**Julie Lusk, MEd, E-RYT,** specializes in balancing and strengthening the body-mind-spirit connection through yoga, meditation, therapeutic relaxation, and guided imagery. With more than thirty years of experience, she is an internationally published author whose books include *Yoga Meditations*. Lusk is president of Wholesome Resources, which provides workshops, retreats, engaging articles, and resource materials on stress management, wellness promotion, yoga, and mind-body techniques and strategies for personal and professional growth to thrive in today's world.

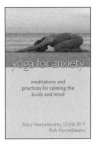
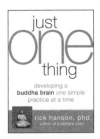
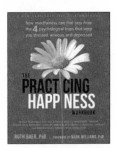
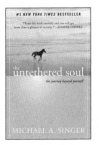
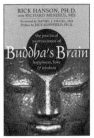
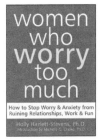

Register your **new harbinger** titles for additional benefits!

When you register your **new harbinger** title—purchased in any format, from any source—you get access to benefits like the following:

- Downloadable accessories like printable worksheets and extra content

- Instructional videos and audio files

- Information about updates, corrections, and new editions

Not every title has accessories, but we're adding new material all the time.

Access free accessories in 3 easy steps:

1.  Sign in at NewHarbinger.com (or **register** to create an account).

2.  Click on **register a book**. Search for your title and click the **register** button when it appears.

3.  Click on the **book cover or title** to go to its details page. Click on **accessories** to view and access files.

That's all there is to it!

If you need help, visit:

NewHarbinger.com/accessories

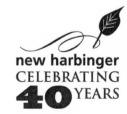

**new harbinger**
CELEBRATING
**40** YEARS